To Pamela

Pennye Lente

Based on a True Story

IN REMISSION
A Family's Struggle to Save Their Beloved Dog

PENNYE A. LENTES

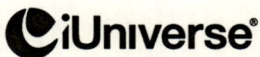

IN REMISSION
A FAMILY'S STRUGGLE TO SAVE THEIR BELOVED DOG

Copyright © 2014 Pennye A. Lentes.

All rights reserved. No part of this book may be used or reproduced by any means, graphic, electronic, or mechanical, including photocopying, recording, taping or by any information storage retrieval system without the written permission of the publisher except in the case of brief quotations embodied in critical articles and reviews.

iUniverse books may be ordered through booksellers or by contacting:

iUniverse
1663 Liberty Drive
Bloomington, IN 47403
www.iuniverse.com
1-800-Authors (1-800-288-4677)

Because of the dynamic nature of the Internet, any web addresses or links contained in this book may have changed since publication and may no longer be valid. The views expressed in this work are solely those of the author and do not necessarily reflect the views of the publisher, and the publisher hereby disclaims any responsibility for them.

Any people depicted in stock imagery provided by Thinkstock are models, and such images are being used for illustrative purposes only.
Certain stock imagery © Thinkstock.

ISBN: 978-1-4917-5153-4 (sc)
ISBN: 978-1-4917-5154-1 (hc)
ISBN: 978-1-4917-5155-8 (e)

Printed in the United States of America.

iUniverse rev. date: 12/04/2014

Dedication

To my husband, John, whose compassion and continued dedication to keeping Ms. Piggy in remission was integral in her staying strong and in our lives for as long as possible.

And to Kermit, who seemed to know how sick she was and always took a backseat instead of wanting the same amount of attention from us.

To my readers and fellow dog lovers. Enjoy the book and our stories. Here's a picture of Piggy enjoying her favorite place on the deck.

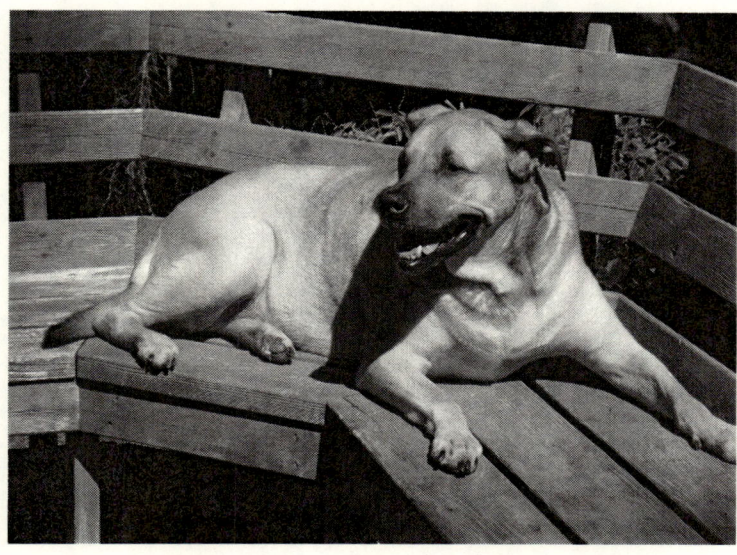

Acknowledgments

Dr. Annie Theissan, DVM (and the devoted staff at Chambers Creek Veterinarian Clinic in Lakewood, Washington). Her caring nature, confidence, and support made it possible for us to weather the toughest of times while Ms. Piggy endured six months of chemotherapy. Annie knew Piggy from the time she was eight weeks old and saw her through a variety of health problems.

I want to publicly say thank you to Betty, my mother-in-law, for everything she did as I tried to recuperate from painful surgeries. She helped take care of not only me but her "grandpups" too. And, as you can see, she loves both of them very much.

Many thanks to Cindy at REI (Recreational Equipment, Inc.), who spoke up and led us in the right direction in a time of confusion, sadness, and turmoil! And to Rhonda, who knew and understood the kind of love we had for Piggy.

Many thanks to the manager at the Sumner, Washington, Feed and Grain Store for turning us on to this food! He stayed late to help me that night and told me some success stories surrounding this particular brand of food that gave me reasons to believe we could save our Piggy.

Dr. Sarah Gillings, DVM, DACVIM, of Summit Referral Center. It seemed like a sign from up above that Dr. Gillings and her associates moved to Tacoma from Seattle to open up a center full of specialists devoted to canine and feline cancer within a couple of weeks of Piggy finishing her chemo at Chambers Creek.

Introduction

As I sit here on the deck, my mind drifts back to December 5, 2009, and the tremendous fortune we have been blessed with over the past three years. Our dog, Ms. Piggy, had been diagnosed with lymphoma. Doc Annie (our favorite veterinarian) said, "She will be gone within a month if you decide against any further treatment." We believed this, because one day she just stopped eating and continued to have no interest in food. (Remember this if your pet suddenly makes a major change in eating habits; get to the vet as soon as possible.)

Some people might not understand our deep feelings for Ms. Piggy, but she was our four-legged princess and meant the world to us. The veterinarian stressed to us, "There are no guarantees. Even with aggressive treatment, you might buy only an additional year of quality life." But Ms. Piggy was only seven years old. She still had so much life left to live, even if some people would consider her just a pet.

We barely had enough money to make our mortgage, let alone start chemotherapy that might run as much as $6,000. We were just starting to get caught up on our credit card bills. We didn't think more than a moment before making the decision. Within two days, we began six months of intense efforts to save her life.

I had a credit card called Care Credit that I had used for some major dental work; to our surprise, it was for vet bills too. The terms of this credit card can be negotiated based on the doctor's, dentist's, or veterinarian's office. Working with Chambers Creek, we were able to use this card without interest if it was paid off in less than twelve months. We eliminated all expenses that weren't absolutely essential. We even reduced the size and frequency of our trash pickups (with only two people, we never filled our containers up anyway) and changed to bimonthly versus every-week pickup. It turned out this was all we really needed anyway, so we have kept it this way.

While taking Pigs for her weekly blood tests and chemo, I met more and more people in the same situation. I enjoyed sharing information about Piggy's progress. I'd start conversations to pass along any helpful details we might have discovered during our research with the hope of receiving some new ideas in return. I realized how many people needed support and help in dealing with this illness. I met men who were reduced to tears when they realized their longtime pet—a real member of the family—had some form of cancer.

I kept a journal of our struggles, successes, and failures. The addition of a great all-natural diet helped keep her in remission and in our lives for almost three more years. I'm sorry to say she came out of remission and passed on December 4, 2012, but we relished every single day we were given. Our initial expectations were gaining an extra year with her, but instead she was healthy and full of life for almost three more years. It was worth every single sacrifice we made.

With this book, I hope to give others a reason to believe in a treatment that can extend the lives of their four-legged best friends for much longer than they might think. Since the diagnosis, we've discovered information on the harmful aspects of many foods on the market today and the value of a true high-protein, high-fat (yes, high fat!), all-natural, and nutrient-packed grain-free meal plan. I've included recipes for the diet we used and suggested supplements and natural remedies for possible side effects brought on by the chemo drugs.

I hope you find this book helpful whether you're dealing with an illness with a family member or your precious pet. It's a heartwarming story that taught me there's always hope, no matter how desperate the situation may seem. I can't make any promises my suggestions will work for you, but they will give you a major head start. We did a large amount of research before making the decision to totally change our dogs' diets. We continued to feed Kermit our special diet, hoping to hang on to him for a long time to come. He joined Ms. Piggy much sooner than we had hoped. Is there a dog heaven? I hope so.

Chapter One

Move after Move

We made our big move from southern Florida across the country to Washington State in the year 2000. Florida single-family homes with decent-sized yards were out of our price range, and we weren't allowed to have any pets in the condo we rented. (Although, my husband did have a python named Monty. Snakes didn't really fall into the standard "pet" category, so we were able to keep him. I mean, how much of a mess does a snake really make?) But now that we had moved, it was a different story.

My thirteen-year-old son had decided to go and live with his father (my ex) in the Midwest. I was heartbroken. Unfortunately, in the state where he was born (and where my first marriage ended) the child is allowed at the age of thirteen to decide which parent they want to live with. I probably could have won a custody battle—I had a good job, was in the process of remarrying, and was his biological mother—but I felt he would resent me for the rest of his life if I forced him to stay.

While living in Florida, I'd had two employers over an eight-year period and spent about three years at each job. When my current job was eliminated because of an acquisition and an inevitable merging of positions, there really weren't any other jobs available in the area. I took a part-time position while looking for a more permanent one.

We decided that, with all of the changes in our lives, we should pursue a fresh start away from Florida. A potential employer flew my husband and me to the Seattle area. The weather was 70 degrees, Mount Rainier was intoxicating, and we felt our interviews went well. It seemed like everything was falling into place and this move was meant to be—like we were headed to heaven on earth, with a little rain in the mix.

A couple of weeks later we made the decision to move completely across the country, and thus began a new chapter of our lives. New doesn't always mean better. I guess this is kind of like the saying that the grass isn't always greener on the other side of the pasture. The weather was okay, although sometimes a little too wet. But property with a little land in Washington was much more affordable, and we knew we would soon be able to have a home with a large enough backyard for a dog or maybe even two.

John and I packed up our belongings and hired a moving company. We were given an estimate of three weeks for delivery of our belongings. Then we rented a U-Haul large enough to take a month's worth of anything we might need for the trip, clothes for the next three or four weeks, and Monty, my husband's snake. John was not about to ship Monty with any reptile shipping company, no matter how reputable they were. We devised a plan (I say "we" but John should receive credit for the plan) to put Monty's large tank in the U-Haul so we'd have it available as soon as we arrived, but we'd keep Monty with us in the Jeep in a smaller tank for the drive to Washington and for ease of carrying him in and out of hotels along the way. We snuck him in the back entrances of the hotels and kept him in the room closets with a cover over the cage during the trip. Snakes are nocturnal, so I'm sure this messed with his internal time clock just like the change in time zones messed with ours.

The first real kink in our plan occurred when we decided to stay over at my mom's house as we passed through the Midwest. We wanted to stay a day or so and visit my son and the rest of the family. John took Monty to the bedroom closet and got him settled for the night. We didn't think about asking Mom if it was okay. I really didn't think he would be seen by anyone. He was safely confined and couldn't get loose, so what was the harm? We went back out to the U-Haul and pulled out the few plants we'd brought and watered them for the next leg of the trip.

When we were finished, we went inside to talk to my mom and let her know Monty was in the closet. She laughed and thought we were joking. We said again, "No, really—Monty is in the closet," and we assured her that we weren't kidding. She didn't look very happy. She said she didn't think she'd be able to sleep in the same house as a snake. I felt bad that I hadn't cleared it with her ahead of time. I guess no matter what your age, lessons can always be learned. (My dad, who has passed away, had quite a dry sense of humor. I'm not sure whether or not he was laughing as he looked down at this exchange from heaven.) My nieces and nephews all wanted to see the snake, but I don't think this helped reduce my mom's desire to sleep elsewhere for the night. In the end, we convinced her that Monty was harmless. One of my nephews wanted some snakeskin and asked if we could save it the next time Monty shed and send it to him. Later that year, I sent it to him. I think he took it to show-and-tell at school. My nephew's excitement was a bright spot in what would turn out to be a very rough trip across the country.

Just a note to anyone who is driving across the country from the southern tip of Florida to the northern tip of Washington State: it's more stressful than planning a wedding. I was beginning to think only one of us might make it to Washington alive. When we finally arrived fourteen days later, we were barely speaking to each other. It was very late in the evening, and we were both scheduled to begin our new jobs the next day. *Bummer!* I just wanted a good night's sleep. Instead, I was looking at sleeping on a carpeted floor with a sleeping bag for a mattress for more nights than I cared to think about.

We rented for the first couple of years to give us time to decide what area near Tacoma we'd best like to live. We wanted to be fairly close to work but gave the real estate agent a pretty broad radius for the initial search We made sure there was a spare bedroom just in case Jason decided to come and live with us. Arranging for a place to live from the other side of the country (without meeting someone in person) had been difficult. Luckily, we had been able to take a virtual tour of the area close to the apartment we were looking at renting. But we couldn't tour the actual apartments available, and there were only a few complexes that would agree to rent to us without a face-to-face interview. We found a decent-sized apartment to rent with a one-year lease. I wasn't really keen on staying in an apartment for that long, but it was something I had to deal with because we had only one month to pack up and finalize a place to live. In the end, we had only fourteen days to completely relocate across country. The only thought that kept me going throughout this process was that in a year we could purchase a home of our own and actually have a big yard.

My son was still with my ex husband in Missouri. When he was thirteen (legal age in MO to decide), he chose to move from Florida back with his father to attend high school. I was heartbroken so I through myself in to work and held out hope he would like Washington better than Florida when he came for holidays and summer vacations it would become permanent. We were in a great school district in Tacoma and would be a great addition to the Curtis High School football team. As it turned out, he changed his mind and decided to stay with his father and finish high school in Missouri. Although, he visited and I kept tabs on his progress by keeping in close contact with my family which totaled over twenty five and at the time included my mom, six siblings, multiple nieces, nephews and many friends and in-laws. When I look back now it might seem like I was trying to replace my son with a dog but I still had high hopes he would join us in Washington and we would be all be a great family including John and I, my son and a rescued dog.

Every time I saw someone walking or running with their dog, I grew more and more impatient for having one myself. I grew up with a hound dog named Sam. My brothers and I used to sit with Sam on the steps in the backyard. We would look into the sky and make a howling noise that sounded kind of like a wolf, and Sam would howl along with us. It seemed funny back then, but now I realize he was howling because it was hurting his ears.

Buying a house is a big decision. We wanted to be located in a nice area and have plenty of space in our yard. When our apartment lease was coming to an end, we tried to decide where we wanted to live permanently. We wanted a fairly large home with a yard in a specific neighborhood, located in the suburbs of Tacoma. We decided to wait another year to buy a home to give us time to save for a bigger down payment. Fortunately, we found a small house for rent in the area we wanted to eventually buy and live. At least we wouldn't have to stay in an apartment for another year. The bad news was there were no pets allowed. But the good news was, my son was coming to live with us again. We gave him the upstairs loft in the rental home. My son seemed to go back and forth to Missouri more times that I can count but in the end he was a graduate of Curtis High School. The year after graduation he spent working for the Economic Development Department and earned a $5,000 tuition scholarship for leadership and service.

One year later, we were finally in a position to buy the kind of home we wanted. We began looking. The downturn in the housing market hadn't begun yet, so homes were still at a fairly high market value and even higher based on the type of neighborhood where we were looking. And then it happened. In May 2002, we discovered the perfect home for us. It was scheduled for an open house the day after we first saw it. Luckily, our real estate agent had found out about it ahead of time and was able to get the key to show us around. It was Memorial Day. Though it was only about the fifth house we had looked at, we knew from the minute we walked inside and stepped out on the huge deck that this was the one for us. This house had a three-tiered backyard, a basketball court, and even a large, covered dog kennel. We hadn't even considered a kennel as a requirement or asset when looking at other listings. It was almost like it was our destiny to rescue a dog. Kind of like kismet. We were destined to have a dog.

By late June 2002, we were finally moved in and had a home that was perfect for owning a dog. We couldn't believe it already had a large, covered outdoor kennel and the backyard was completely enclosed with a six-feet-tall wood fence. The backyard had three entrances. That made it seem like a fortress, but one that would come in handy for more that the most obvious reasons—and one in particular that would last for many years to come. I just knew there had to be one of the most perfect dogs calling out our name and begging to be part of our family. We spent six months getting settled in and waited until December before seriously thinking about looking for a dog. We were a little worried about house-training during the winter, but we were so excited we just couldn't wait.

Chapter Two
Becoming a Pet Owner

It was a given that we would rescue a dog from our local Humane Society. I recommend this to anyone wanting to add a furry friend to their family. We tried to think through any problems that might arise so we could be prepared from the very beginning. With both of us working during the day, we didn't want to leave the dog in the outside kennel during the colder, rainy months. We wanted to have plenty of play time after work and during the weekends. We thought we'd gone through any possible troubles and addressed them ahead of time. We knew it would be really quiet now that my son had moved back to live with his father again soon after completing his year with the Economic Development Department. We were very proud of him and had hopes he would use his scholarship for training. We decided it was the ideal timing for that perfect dog now that once again, we had become empty nesters.

Lesson one for any of you who are considering adopting a cat or dog: there's always something that didn't make the preparation list—some little (or big) detail you didn't think about because you were too excited about the blessed event. Be ready for anything and everything.

Here is a checklist of considerations you might want to have a handle on before you adopt your pet:

1. If you rescue a dog, you will most likely be required to spay or neuter him/her if it hasn't already been done. Most places

will share the cost or give you a reduced rate. Some will automatically implant a tracking chip in case your pet gets lost.
2. There are many different types of needs based on the gender, age, and breed of pet, which you should consider before you decide on a new pet. For example, some require more exercise (depending on age and breed), and it's better to have space for larger breeds vs. apartment-style living.
3. Do you have children at home? This should be taken into consideration when choosing breed, gender, and the reasons the animal was in the shelter to begin with. A sad story we encountered was a nine-year-old very large breed who had been with the same family since birth. It was given up because the family had a baby and was worried the dog would be harmful. The reason I even mention this is so you think ahead to any foreseeable lifestyle changes that would cause you to surrender your pet to a shelter. I have many stories similar to this (we are near an air force/army base) but none quite as sad.
4. You will need a crate, but take into consideration the full-grown size of the dog you plan on adopting before you purchase one. We purchased an extra-large crate that would accommodate both dogs until they were a couple of months older. They bonded and snuggled with each other every night. When it became evident that they required their own personal space, we purchased a second identical one. (After being side by side during the night, we didn't want them to be scared or lonely. The sides of the kennels were solid, and so my husband came up with the most loving solution. He used his Dremel to cut one- to two-inch holes down the sides of both kennels so the dogs could always see each other. How sweet is that!) I highly recommend house-training with the crate method, but you must be committed to this from the start if you get a puppy or an outside dog.
5. Be prepared for chewing. We didn't have this problem, but I made sure the dogs always had fresh bones with marrow to keep them occupied while we were at work during the day. Excessive chewing doesn't usually go on forever, rather just as they are getting their permanent teeth (kind of like a baby).

6. Get a decent small-sized carpet shampooer. No matter how good your dog's training is, you will be glad to have it. The faster you catch accidents, the better.
7. During house-training particularly, try to find a way to come home once a day for a potty break. I had an hour lunch, so I used this time to run home. Other options becoming more popular in today's world are doggy day cares and people who walk dogs for a living. If you are going to be gone for any extended period of time, be prepared to pay to kennel your pet. (We could never bring ourselves to do this.)
8. Depending on the anticipated full-grown size of your pet, it is nice to have a vehicle to accommodate them. We had a Jeep Cherokee prior to rescuing our dogs, so it worked out for us to rescue larger breeds. When we traded up, it was a no-brainer when we picked our Ford Explorer. SUVs also came in handy for trips to the beach or mountains and for camping. This also helps the dog get used to going to the vet and they are more likely to become less fearful with every visit. Many places that offer grooming, trim nails as a part of the package.
9. Be prepared to handle an accident or illness. Having pets is just like having a child except one with two more legs. Some breeds are more prone to specific diseases (for example, labs are more likely to have allergies and skin rashes and some larger breeds are more likely to have tumors). We didn't find this out until a few years after our adoption.
10. Many animals don't like their nails clipped. (We have one of those.) There are many ways to handle this, depending on the degree of fear. You can use tranquilizers that need to be administered from one to two hours prior to your vet visit. It also helps to cover the animal's eyes or, as a last resort, put a muzzle on them. The muzzle is really to protect the person who is clipping the nails from getting bitten. Last but not least, get nails clipped on a regular basis, which also helps ensuring regular visits and checkups.

Having pets is a lot like having children. They can be involved in an accident or get sick at the drop of a hat, so be prepared. If you travel, you'll need to be ready to put them in a kennel or have

In Remission

someone lined up to sit with them. If you get a young puppy, it will whine or cry for attention during the middle of the night because it's missing its mother. Be prepared for your pet wanting to sleep with you too.

    I want to say that up front that even though there are some negatives, (speaking from experience) there are more positives. As you read on, prepare for some of the best and most heartwarming "dog tales" you've ever heard.

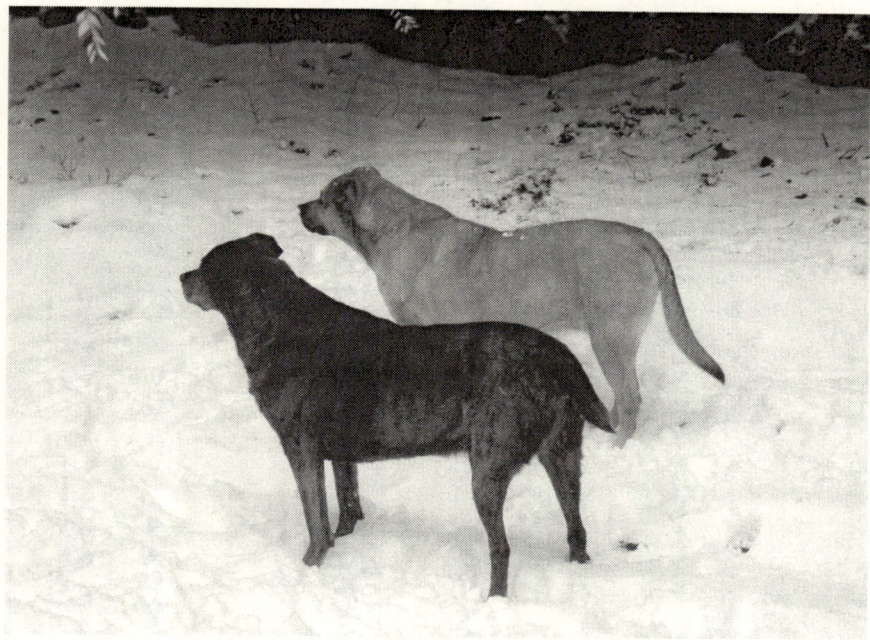

(dogs in snow)

Chapter Three

The Adoption

We made our first trip to the Pierce County Humane Society just before Christmas to see what kinds of dogs were available for adoption. The first one that caught my eye was a mastiff mix. He curled up behind John's legs when we stepped into the section where he was being housed. It was almost as if he picked us. He was about ten weeks old, had a cropped tail, and was a beautiful brindle (black/brown) color. He had wrinkly skin on his face and was a bit shy, but I was in love with him already. We could tell he was scared of almost everything, including other dogs and most humans. The signs of past abuse were evident. As soon as he curled up behind John's legs, we looked at each other and knew he had to be ours. Surely we could nurture him back to normalcy and he'd become a happy part of our family.

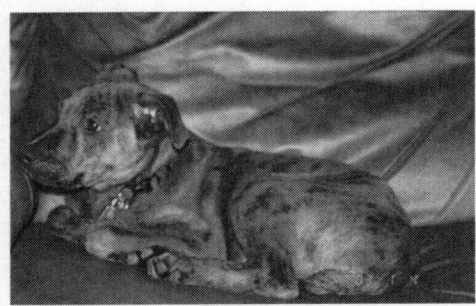
(Kermit as a pup sitting in grey chair)

It was sad to see some of the dogs that had been left at the Humane Society. There was one very large breed dog. He must have been at least 150 pounds, if not more. The workers told us he was nine years old and his owners were having their first baby and didn't trust the dog around children. It didn't seem fair that they could just discard him like that. For anyone looking to adopt or rescue a pet, make sure you want him (or her) for the rest of the pet's life. A pet is not a toy that can be thrown away when the new wears off. It's almost like a marriage. "For better or worse ..."

John and I had discussed whether or not to adopt more than one dog. We decided if we adopted two puppies, then they could enjoy playing with each other while we were at work during the day. We went to put our names at the top of the list for adopting the mastiff mix and look for an additional dog.

We were told the dogs would need to be kept for the required three-day waiting period before they could be adopted. The three-day wait was designed to give the original owners time to claim the animals and also to make sure they are healthy before giving them to a new, loving home. This was when we realized someone could come and claim him during these three days and he might never have a chance at a good life. Whoever had mistreated this dog up to this point didn't deserve to have him back. I prayed he would be ours. As we went in search of another dog to rescue, the waiting began.

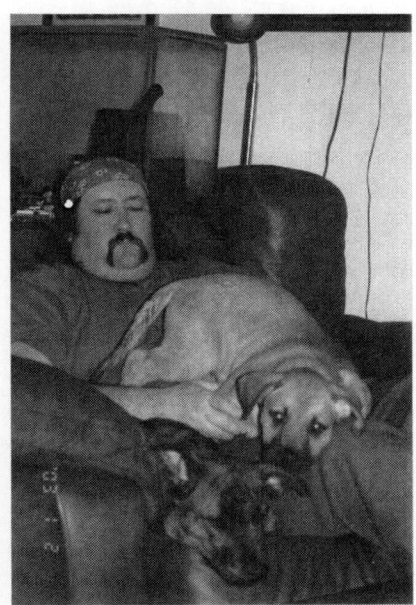

(John & dogs in chair)

We set out to find his lifelong playmate. I heard "someone" barking on the other side of the building, so I headed in that direction. As I rounded a corner, I saw the cutest black-and-tan female puppy jumping up and down as if she was saying, "Pick me, pick me! Please get me out of here." I motioned to John to come over my way.

Almost from the moment he spotted her, I could tell his heart had melted. At around eight weeks old, this shepherd mix seemed to be a little younger and smaller than the mastiff. I said, "Oh, John, we have to have her too." John agreed. That quickly we'd decided to add two new members to our household. Little did I know that she would become John's little princess, having him wrapped around her paw in no time at all. Again, we signed our name to the three-day list and started the waiting process for both dogs. We didn't worry about them getting along. This might have been an oversight on our part, but luckily they seemed like they were meant to be together from the start.

When talking to the people at the Humane Society about our choices, they told us that these two puppies had been left outside in the cold without any type of identification. We drove back home filled with excitement about the dogs we had picked out.

By this time, our son was almost eighteen. He would soon be leaving for college or his declared career and then would be out on his own. As (almost) empty nesters, we needed these dogs almost as much as they needed us.

We researched the two breeds on the Internet and realized both dogs were going to be quite large when full grown. This didn't matter. We had a large, fenced-in backyard, and our house included a full finished basement with a large entertainment room perfect for their first home base. A set of sliding glass doors led out from our daylight basement to the backyard and the outdoor kennel. It was going to be just perfect!

We started getting ready for the dogs with the hopes no one would go to the Humane Society to claim them during the next three days. One of our first purchases was an extra-large carrier/kennel. We thought they could sleep together at night while they were still puppies, creating a permanent bond—just like siblings. Had we thought through every teeny, tiny possible problem, we might have bought two crates in the beginning in case it took them time to get used to one another. (We planned on buying a matching one as they grew larger and needed more room to themselves.) But, luckily, when we removed Kermit from the extremely loud and crowded Humane Society kennel he was in, his fear subsided. The dogs seemed to love each other almost immediately.

In the Humane Society, dogs were separated by size and age. Kermit was tall, and to the untrained eye he looked like he could have been three to four months old. As a result, he had been placed in a group of ten to fifteen older dogs in an overcrowded pen. Piggy was a couple of weeks younger than him and was a little shorter. She had this bubbly puppy personality. There were quite a few dogs her size in the same pen; they all seemed to be playing well together. The bond these two dogs were about to create would be one that lasted forever, as if they were truly brother and sister.

We bought large breed puppy dry food, collars, leashes, food bowls for each of them, plus a larger bowl for water. Since we had stairs leading to the basement, we also bought a baby gate to keep them from falling down the stairs or climbing up them, depending on the time of day and where we wanted them to stay.

This was over the Christmas and New Year's holidays, so the three-day waiting period seemed like eternity. We didn't have any family that lived close to us, so it was just the three of us. We were nervous that someone would come in to claim the dogs. (Although, anyone who would abandon them out in the cold without a collar really didn't deserve to get them back.)

On day four, we were ready to pick up our new additions. As soon as we got the call from the Humane Society, we loaded up the pet carrier and headed to pick up our new son and daughter. We had made all kinds of plans, such as how we would house-train them, where they would be allowed to go, and so on. The list of rules and regulations seemed endless.

We arrived at the Humane Society and waited in line for our turn. When we got to the head of the line, the worker took us to the back of the building. The dogs had been in two different parts of the kennel, so this would be the first time they would meet each other.

This is also where we would watch them implant microchips. If the dogs ever got lost and were picked up, they could be identified with their unique number. Microchips are very common these days. They are implanted usually in the back of the neck. When an animal is brought to an animal shelter, the microchip can be read with a small handheld gun. The chip is linked to a database that includes the owner's name, address, and phone number. The chip number is also registered with the local police. The implantation process was quick and easy, and we were assured it was painless. Our hope was that these numbers would follow them all of their lives and protect them from harm or getting lost.

Once we were done with all of the paperwork, we brought them, one by one, out to the crate in the back of our Jeep. First, I brought Kermit. He seemed subdued and scared. When I came back with Piggy, Kermit backed up in the crate and made room for her. They sniffed each other and then started licking one another's ears (one of the ways a dog shows affection). They were so cute, cuddling and playing together almost from the beginning. It seemed like they had known each other for all of their short lives. Kermit was kind of timid at first, but Piggy was jumping around and eventually got Kermit to be a little more playful. It took him a little longer to warm up to her and to us. This was the start of their lives together. Little did they know it, but they would go on to spend the next ten years together.

Chapter Four
Settling In

For the most part, our list of rules went out of the window on day one. The dogs both were almost immediately in my husband's lap in his leather La-Z-Boy chair. They began their reign of our hearts and home right away. Now came the difficult task of coming up with names for them. John wanted to call the mastiff Chief. Of course, John wanted what most men would, which was to call him a more masculine name. I looked at John and said, "He's just not a Chief." The male mastiff was kind of goofy as opposed to a leader, timid and shy and anything but a commander. He seemed almost depressed, but we thought he had to be happy to be away from the crowded kennel. John agreed with me about the name, so we continued to try to think of other names that might fit their personalities.

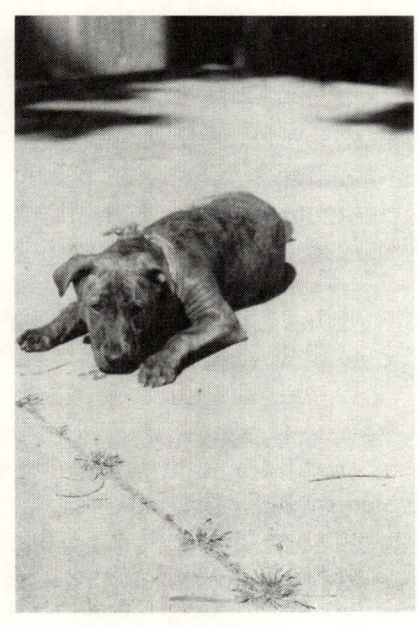

(Kermit on bball court)

The female shepherd mix was a feisty, hyper little dog. She loved to play and lick us in the face and could eat anything and everything put in front of her. This made one of the important rules—no table scraps—hard to follow! As most dogs do, they begged and begged for something off our plates even if they had just eaten dinner. And so her name was born from this characteristic: Piggy. Her name led to my next thought, "He is definitely a Kermit." The dogs fit with each other like two lost souls that had been found and brought together for the greater good. And so they became Kermit and Ms. Piggy Lentes.

No sooner had they learned their names then we came up with half a dozen nicknames for them. For Piggy, we might call out Pigsy, Princess, Pretty Girl, Girly Girl, or my personal favorite, Piggy Pooh.

It became clear that our original suspicions were right—Kermit's previous "parents" were likely abusive. It took him longer to warm up to us. Someone had treated him very badly, even docking his tail the painful way (without visiting a veterinarian). We believe they probably thought he was a Rottweiler, pit bull, or some other kind of purebred and this was the cheapest way to bob the tail. It took him two or three months before he began to wag his tail (what was left of it). I can remember the first time he cautiously emerged from the crate. It took him a while before he stopped flinching when we raised our hand to pet his head. We felt so good that we had adopted him and he would have a great new home. Eventually, he turned into the loving and loyal Kermit. Our funniest nickname for him is Butt Wagger. You see, his rear end is large, and when he wags his tail he moves his whole backside. It's really funny to see him in action. I've heard this is the way purebred mastiffs wag their tails. When he gets excited, his entire back end moves back and forth, faster and faster.

We decided to house-train them using the crate method. When you have two dogs, this way is much easier than other methods. You can feed them at the same time and cut off their water at night at the same time. At the end of the evening, we would let them drink and then go outside to do what we have always called "their business." In the beginning while they were still very little, I got up with them in the middle of the night and let them out. They would give a little *yip yip* from their crate, and I would hear them, wake up, and let them outside. (I was a light sleeper, which made it easier.)

When they got too big to stay in the same crate, we bought an identical large crate and split them up. John was so sweet. He used the Dremel to drill out one- to two-inch holes halfway up the crates. We pushed them close together; this way they could see each other through the holes and keep from getting lonely.

As their bladders got bigger and they learned how to "hold it," we allowed them to start sleeping with us. (*Big mistake!*) They were so loving and always wanted to cuddle up with us. It was hard to resist.

They grew fast and learned very quickly what the words "their business" meant. And yes, they actually slept in our bed for a few months—until they got so big that they took up too much room. We had a king-size bed. Piggy slept between us, and Kermit stretched across the foot. It didn't take long for them to outgrow their spots. (Plus, they were pushing us off the bed.)

When they were about twelve weeks old, we bought a couple of what would be the first of many fluffy beds for them to sleep in on the floor at the foot of our beds. There was still a short period of time we allowed them to sleep in the bed after that, but they outgrew this quickly when they realized how much more room they had on the floor in their own beds. It is just like breaking a child of sleeping with you when they are little and have a bad dream or make up other excuses to sleep in your bed. With cats or dogs, space wouldn't be such a problem with small breeds. (Although, it does cut down on together time for Mom and Dad.) It's one thing if you have a small dog that stays little, but ours weighed over one hundred pounds at one point. Just imagine what that would look like.

Chapter Five

Making Them Part of Our Family

One day, about three weeks after adopting the dogs, I returned home to discover a voice mail message. As I listened, a lump formed in my throat. The call was from the Humane Society. Someone had come to look for their dog and identified one of ours from a picture that was still on their bulletin board. They said they thought it was their dog. The message continued, saying as far as the Humane Society was concerned we were the rightful owners. They said it was up to us if we wanted to contact the possible original owner, whose phone number was given in the message. They didn't tell us whether it was Piggy or Kermit, and at this point I didn't even want to know.

When John came home from work later that day, I told him about the message. By this time, Kermit and Piggy had been ours for more than three weeks. I looked at John and said, "I wonder which one it is." In my heart I knew he would be torn to pieces if it was Piggy, as he had grown so attached to her in the short time she'd been with us. She was his little princess. In the beginning, I felt he would bond with Kermit because he was male and had a mellow, laid-back personality (a lot like John) and Piggy was kind of hyper, like me. It turned out to be just the opposite. Piggy was John's little princess, and Kermit stuck to me like glue. Maybe Kermit liked the maternal way I treated him. I still haven't figured this one out. I thought Piggy and I would be best friends, but from the beginning this gentle smile would come over John's face whenever she was around, no matter what she might be doing. He could never get mad at her. For example, she had a very long tongue. Every time we got in the car, Piggy would sneak up and lick John in the ear. It got to be a running joke. She almost looked as if she was smiling when she did it.

My heart swelled when John said, "I don't care which one it is—we're not giving up either one." Even after seven years of marriage and several huge hurdles, I found a new level of love for John.

We cried together, talked it over, and decided no one who waits three weeks before searching for their missing puppy during the cold of winter deserves to have the dog back. I threw away the note that contained the phone number I had written down from the voice mail. We were already madly in love with Kermit and Piggy, so that was the end of it. We never discussed it again. I have to admit, I did still think about it for quite a while. Part of me wondered if some little girl or boy was missing the puppy they received for Christmas. Maybe, by some big mistake, it had gotten loose and the parents didn't know where to look. But life went on as we enjoyed our new family. Between the dogs and work, we kept busy. As time passed, we knew we'd made the right decision.

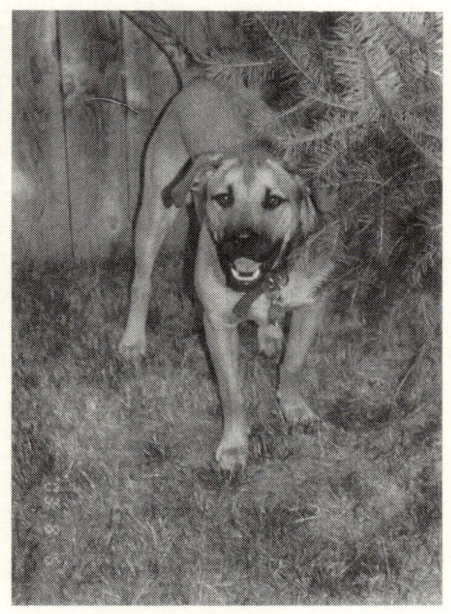

(Piggy)

The dogs were just like a couple of children but with different personalities. They played together like a brother and sister. Sometimes they played rough, and other times they would give each other kisses. Remember that for dogs, a lick in the ear is a sign of affection.

Pennye A. Lentes

When we adopted them from the Humane Society, we signed an agreement that required us to get them spayed and neutered within two months of adoption. I guess this was a reasonable request, to prevent more abandoned puppies down the road. But the puppies were still so little, and I was scared for them to have to go through this surgery. This was when I first realized what a blessing it was that we had done the research and chosen Chambers Creek Veterinary Hospital to handle their care. Their office was pretty close to where we lived, and they had a great reputation.

Our two precious dogs went to Chambers Creek Veterinary Hospital for all health-related checkups and problems—the first being getting them spayed and neutered. I really didn't want to make the dogs go through "getting fixed." Though I worried it would be traumatic and painful for them, I knew it was something I had to do. I was unsure of the recovery time and was concerned about being able to take off work to care for them during the day.

I took the puppies in to the veterinary office early on a Thursday morning in February 2003 and picked them up when I got off work later that day. We were instructed to keep an eye on them for at least the next two to three days to make sure they didn't rip out their stitches by jumping or playing too rough. We thought about separating them, but they followed each other around everywhere. When forced to be apart, they whined for each other. They were confined to the basement at this point, so they didn't try to climb the stairs. Luckily, John was able to take a couple of days off of work so someone could be here with them during the first days following the procedures. At that point in time, it was easier for him rather than me to take off of work. His boss loved animals and had seen the puppies in our truck when we first got them. He was so sweet when John asked for Friday off to take care of them. On the other hand, my boss hated dogs and animals in general. I wanted to say to him that he didn't know what he was missing.

The dogs were such troupers. The day after surgery, they were up and playing like nothing ever happened. By the time the weekend went by and we went back to work on Monday, both of them were up and around, ready to play. We tried to restrain them from jumping, but nothing could keep them down. They acted as if nothing ever happened. I was happy to have this ordeal over and done.

In Remission

All of the veterinarians and assistants would get to know Ms. Piggy and Kermit by name and become aware of any special needs or quirks each of them would develop. For example, Piggy was the lover who would lick all of them in the face whenever she'd get a chance. She always wanted treats and jumped up on the checkout counter for extra attention. Kermit did not play well with others and usually required a muzzle and four people to hold him down when getting his nails trimmed.

We included Kermit and Ms. Piggy in everything we did and took them everywhere we went. If we went to Stevens Pass for a few days of fun in the snow, we had to have a place to stay that accepted pets. (For those of you who aren't familiar with western Washington ski areas, Stevens Pass is a popular ski resorts during the winter months and has terrific bike paths in summer.) It was the same when we went to the beach. Both of them loved both the snow and the beach.

Luckily, Washington State is a pet-friendly place to live. Around 70 percent of the population owns some kind of pet. It never even entered our mind to put the dogs in a kennel when we needed to travel. Unfortunately, Kermit could get kind of dangerous with someone he didn't know, so hiring a pet sitter wasn't an option. We'd take separate vacations so one of us would be at home with the dogs at all times—which, at times, was sort of relaxing. It also caused some hardships. There were a few times when there was a death in one of our families and only one person could go. It would have been nice to have the spouse there for emotional support. Our grandson was born four years ago, and John has only seen pictures. I visit

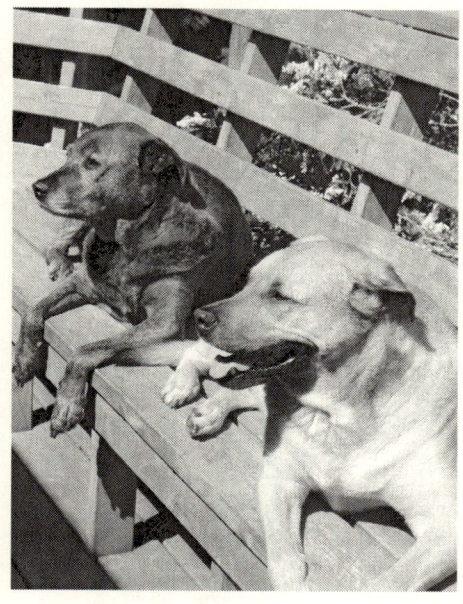

(Dogs enjoying sun on the deck)

once a year for a week by myself. (Our families live in different states in the Midwest.)

However, nothing seemed to beat lying on our deck at home when the sun was bright and the sky was blue. These kinds of days were few and far between in the Seattle area, so we all relished them when they came along. Don't get me wrong, I didn't miss the hundred degree weather and high humidity of Florida, but I could have stood for some warmer weather. I dreamed about retiring to a small house in the Florida Keys with the dogs and couldn't help but picture Kermit swimming in the ocean and Piggy chasing birds on the beach. We can all dream of the ideal retirement, can't we?

Chapter Six

Growing Up

    Both dogs loved the sun, but Piggy Pooh was always more of an outdoors type of dog. Nothing held her back from playing outside or chasing squirrels and birds. We found ways to treat any ailment that came along and did everything we could to make life as normal and fun as it should be, no matter what was going on with her health. Ms. Piggy was always our problem child—allergies, ear infections, and arthritis in her front shoulders while she was still very young.

    Many allergy reactions occur on dogs' feet and between their toes, manifested in a red rash. This is how it was with Ms. Piggy. As a result, she took great care to walk around any grass. We had a basketball court, sandbox, and areas under large trees without grass. She made sure to walk on these areas when she was in the backyard. She had a favorite spot under the middle evergreen tree where it was mainly dirt because the sun couldn't shine through the limbs. When we were looking for her, we could count on finding her there. Even if it was raining, she'd be there. As long as she kept off the grass, her paws wouldn't break out in a rash. Because of this problem, John built a rock path through a grassy area where she liked to walk. The path did enhance the landscape of the backyard, but we know who it was really made for.

    Kermit tended to stick to the inside. It's almost like he was scared to let us out of his sight. He went outside when it was necessary, but he would want right back in after he finished his "business." When it was raining, Kermit looked for a place under the deck or a tree, then he'd run back to the sliders to come back inside. We would have to dry him off right away with a towel or he would rub against the furniture.

The only time his aversion to the outdoors didn't hold true was during trips to the beach or rivers near hotels we stayed at. We made the discovery that he loved to swim. Our Kermit, who never liked to take a bath, was one of the best swimmers. Ms. Piggy loved to play with the water hose and sprinklers. Piggy was part Labrador, so we just assumed she would be the swimmer. She had always liked playing in the little swimming pool we had in the yard, but she would go up only past her knees in the river or ocean.

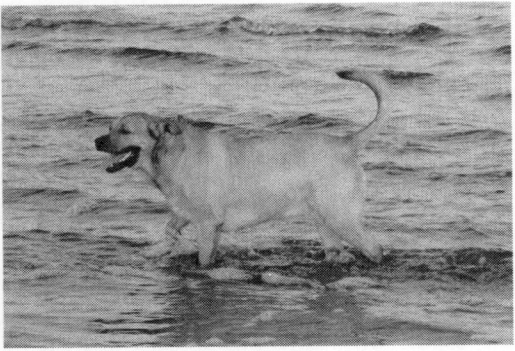

(Piggy in water)

Water play became the best part of our trips. Kermit knew he would get attention when he swam, so as soon as we would hit the ocean or river he'd head for the deepest areas of water and start to swim. We would yell, "Look at Kermit swimming!" over and over as he swam in circles with his head held high. These were some of the rare times when he received more attention than Piggy, because of her health problems. Kermit was our champion swimmer! I felt bad sometimes when Piggy got all of the attention. We had to be painstakingly aware of any changes in her behavior or eating habits. Sometimes I'd forget to buy vitamins or supplements for myself, but I always remembered to get Ms. Piggy's arthritis medication, pay for the week's treatment, or get expensive blood work she might need. It wasn't that we loved one dog more than the other—no, not at all. Piggy just required more care because of her various problems. She would often have stomach issues that required a special diet to resolve. Chicken and rice is easy to digest and gets dogs' systems regular, if you know what I mean. I will not claim that this was my personal miraculous discovery; this was just yet another remedy we had the folks at Chambers Creek to thank for. I understand that many other vets also prescribe this for miscellaneous bathroom problems.

> This is one of the best tips I can give you--chicken and rice can cure many stomach or intestinal problems in canines and many other animals.

Both dogs loved to ride in our Jeep; however, when we decided to purchase a new Ford Explorer in 2004, it was so much better. We felt like royalty driving around. By "we," I mean all four of us—John, Kermit, Ms. Piggy, and most of all, me. When I made the weekly trips to the store, the dogs always came with me. Every time when I'd come out of the store, I would find Kermit in the driver's seat and Piggy in the front passenger seat, just like they were a husband and wife. The Explorer had more room than the Jeep, so we started taking more trips. Long weekends were frequent. John and I would work as hard as we could to enable us to take an extra day or two off or even to leave a little early on Friday. With all of the packing, it was really more worthwhile if we were able to have a three-day weekend, but we stretched it sometimes and just took two long days.

In the summer, we would drive to an out-of-the-way small town called Moclips, Washington, and stay at Hi-Tides Motel. Kermit first learned to swim in the Moclips River. There was a short path from the motel that led to the river. The dogs loved to take this path, which took us from a deeper and wider part of the river to a shallow area with a tall bedrock wall on one side.

When my mother-in-law and Nan (John's grandmother) came to visit, we took them to Moclips. They loved it. When Nan passed away, she wanted a piece of her jewelry buried in the sand. So the next time my mother-in-law visits, we'll be doing this in Nan's memory.

In the winter, we would head to Packwood, Washington, to play in the snow. We stay in a cabin with snow-covered mountains and forests all around. Washington has a huge percentage of pet owners, so pet-friendly places to stay were everywhere. The dogs preferred the beach, probably because of the nice weather and running on the beach. I will always think of dogs as just four-legged people, and this translates into dogs preferring the beach where it's warm.

During one of our first visits to the beach there was a chance of rain, but we didn't want to cancel. We brought along yellow rainsuits and prepared for the worst. We knew the dogs wouldn't care if it was raining as long as they had time on the beach. After arriving at Hi-Tides, we unpacked, put our rainsuits on, and headed to the beach with the dogs. We brought the dog whistles just in case they took off when we let them off leash to run. John and I would get about seventy-five yards apart and let the dogs go, and they would run from one of us to the other. This was our way of training them to listen to us, come when we whistled, and just plain mind us when we called their name. The wind was howling along with the rain, so it wasn't very fun. Then, since the beach was empty, we let them run a little farther. Soon we realized they were out of control. They looked back at us and took off running as fast as they could. We called and whistled, but with the rain, wind, and waves splashing they couldn't (or just didn't want to) hear us. They kept running. We could barely see them through the rain, and we were running as fast as we could. It's not easy running in heavy yellow rainsuits! When they finally stopped, we put them back on the leash and scolded them. Piggy's tongue was hanging out like she was laughing at us, but it was probably just because she was tired from running. We learned many valuable lessons that day: Primarily, the dogs needed more training before letting them off leash in a large area where they could get away. Second, don't try to run in yellow rainsuits. We worked with them in our backyard and in other small fenced-in places near our home. It wasn't long before they listened to the whistles and our voices and we could trust them off leash.

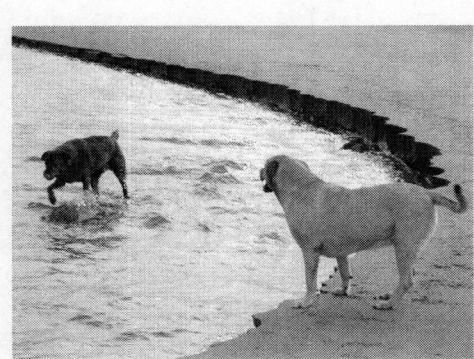

(Kermit and Piggy at beach)

Another reason I know the dogs loved warm weather better was because of their love of our deck. Each of them has their own favorite spot. Piggy liked the corner, where she could curl up and watch the neighbor's kids in their backyard. Kermit liked the floor of the deck, where he could stretch out. For some reason, bumble bees fascinated him. One time they got the best of him. When he came inside from the deck, his eye was almost swollen shut. We rushed him to the vet, and they discovered he had gotten stung. The vet made sure the stinger was gone and there wasn't any damage done to his eye. He had to take prednisone for a few days but was fine.

As I mentioned before, my boss at this time didn't care for my newfound interest in our dogs. He hated the pictures I had in my office because they would always be a conversation piece during meetings. Even outside vendors would ask how the dogs were doing. In the beginning, the dogs provided a good ice breaker for dry topics. When I realized my boss was getting mad, I tried to stop talking about them completely. This realization came when he stated in an open meeting that the only pet he allowed his children to have was a rat (I think he meant a hamster) and it stayed in the garage. But it was too late. People would always ask about the dogs. He'd give me a look that could cut right through me, and I would try to divert to another topic of conversation. I really didn't want to anger my boss. It's not like I started these conversations on purpose or anything; the subject just came up, like when you have a new baby or your child gets their first tooth. Eventually I became nervous when anyone asked me questions about the dogs in front of my boss. I was still running home during my lunch hour to take the dogs out, so this added to the tension. I really don't know where his dislike of animals came from. Looking back, I feel sorry for him. He missed out on so much fun and the love they can add to any family.

Once, another manager got a puppy. He snuck into my office, closed the door and shades, and proceeded to show me the cutest picture of a golden lab. I knew then that the subject was taboo in the office. He must have heard complaints when I wasn't in the room. It's not like the discussions about the dogs were keeping me from getting my job done. I worked very hard and made positive changes in our marketing plans that others were afraid to even mention.

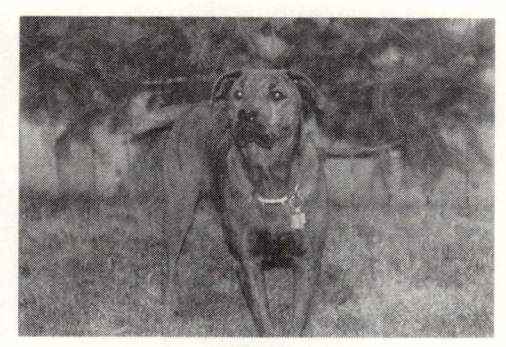

(Kermit)

Pennye A. Lentes

The day in February 2005 when I lost my job turned out to be one of the best days of my life. Although I didn't realize it at that time, it would give me freedom I had never known. No more stress-filled ten-hour days or people pulling at me to produce more and more reports and documentation. Better than that, I could be at home with the dogs while looking for another job. I contemplated even trying to find work I could do from my home office. It was an adventure at first, but little by little I got to the point where I hated to get out of bed in the morning. I guess this might have been a little depression setting in. Kermit and Piggy were the only things that kept me going.

I looked for a new job throughout the next few months but didn't find anything permanent that fit my skill set. I performed some consulting work from home to bring in income. Then in November that same year, after months of doctor visits because of pain in my wrist, I was diagnosed with a rare bone disease. It's called Kienböck's disease and causes the bones in one wrist to shatter. The only bit of silver lining was that it affected my left wrist and I was right handed. Although this disease only affects one wrist, I couldn't believe how hard it was to do things with one hand.

A couple of painful surgeries followed the diagnosis. The first, in December 2005, was an attempt to replace and promote growth of my wrist bones by removing a section of my forearm and placing it where my wrist bones were. The second, in November 2007, removed the half of the bones that hadn't responded to the first attempt and were now dead. As I was recuperating from each of the surgeries, Kermit and Piggy would come to the side of the bed and lick my good hand. I could almost hear them saying, "How are you feeling?" and "I love you." The dogs slept with me in a separate bedroom during this time. They would jump up on the bed, being very careful not to get near my cast. It was as if they were protecting me. Bless John for his patience during this time. The dogs know he was the only one who could let them out downstairs, so they would wait patiently for him to come home.

Although it might sound kind of weird, this disease was another blessing in disguise. I have always been skeptical of this phrase, but if you look at trials in the right way and search for that silver lining, you can find the blessing. And no, I'm not some kind of saint. I only think this way when there's absolutely no other way to process a situation. I didn't realize this was a blessing until December 2009. If it hadn't been for the dogs, my husband, and my mother-in-law, I don't know where I would be today. My mother-in-law dropped everything and came out for a week when I had the surgery. It's weird how quickly the dogs would warm up to her, even after not seeing her for sometimes two or three years. They didn't even do that with some of my friends. That goes to show you what a good judge of character animals can be.

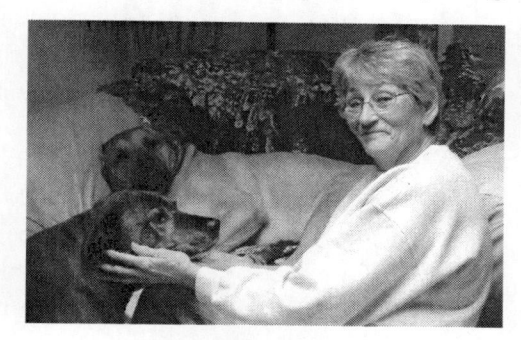

(Kermit, Piggy, Betty)

After the second surgery, I struggled to reinvent myself. I did odd jobs and volunteered at miscellaneous jobs until my wrist would hurt so bad I couldn't do them anymore. I can't describe the degree of loss I felt when I first realized I may never work again, let alone in my field of expertise. I can still remember watching a *Dr. Phil* episode where he urged the unemployed to reinvent themselves in the face of such a horrible economy and high unemployment rate.

The beginning of my transformation was partially out of desperation and somewhat due to our financial circumstances. I continued to compensate for the pain and loss of movement in my left wrist by relying on my right hand heavily and utilizing word recognition software on my computer to type. One of the things that got me through this terrible time was that I never felt alone when I was at home. Kermit and Piggy were always there with me. My husband was supportive in his own way too. He took on a whole new important and hectic role in our household.

I talk to my dogs. The neighbors probably think there's a crazy person living here. Any given day, they could hear me calling to Piggy when she wouldn't come back inside. I'd be yelling, "Piggy Pooh, where are you?" and then she'd come out from behind the garden shed or the bushes. Then as she walked toward me, I'd ask her, "What are you doing?" or "Where have you been?" (Like she was going to answer me.) Kermit was always close to me, so I'd usually be talking to him inside the house. The other day, we (Kermit and I) were watching TV. I said to Kermit, "Oh my gosh—did you see that?" If anyone would have been within earshot and heard this conversation, he or she would have thought I was a crazy lady.

Sometimes I made fun of the dogs. I guess I thought, *They really don't know what I'm saying, so what's the harm?* But after a while, Kermit could tell if I was talking about or making fun of him, and he'd start barking at me. It's almost like he was telling me to stop. Piggy would just come up and start licking me when I laughed at her.

John informed me that I needed to wean Kermit off of the TV shows. (Like that was going to happen.) A few weeks ago, I was recording a movie for Kermit. John had to delete it to make room on our DVR for his recordings. I had to remind him that we must all make sacrifices for the good of the dogs!

The dogs started out sleeping in their crates, but they would whine to get out and get into bed with us. At first they needed help jumping up. After a couple of months, they both had their places and slept with us until they were too big. Then we bought them large dog beds and placed them at the foot of our bed so they'd be close.

When it was hot outside and they were in the backyard, they liked to dig holes and lay in the sandbox. I guess the sand underneath the top layer was cool and felt good. They would jump up all of a sudden and start play fighting or dashing back and forth as fast as they could in the yard. John and I would pretend we were chasing them, and it made them run that much faster.

One day the gate to the backyard was left open, and they escaped to the open road. I started chasing them on foot but soon realized I needed to get the car. I ran back, got their leashes, and hopped in the car to find them. I finally found them five blocks away and convinced them to get in the car. We were careful not to make that mistake again!

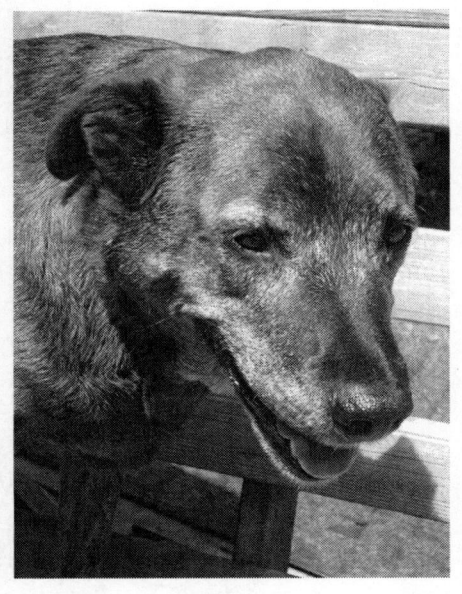

(Kermit)

Chapter Seven

Part 1
Personalities: Ms. Piggy

Piggy was feisty and hyper, and she liked to play with us and with Kermit. She loved looking at herself in the mirror, which she started doing when was she was just a puppy.

At first, Kermit didn't want any part of this. But as he grew a little older, he warmed up to playing in the sandbox and wrestling with Piggy. She turned him from a laid-back, slow-moving dog into the playful one that he is today. Piggy didn't mind change. She'd usually be up for just about anything. I think this helped her make it through some of the toughest days and still come out wagging her tail.

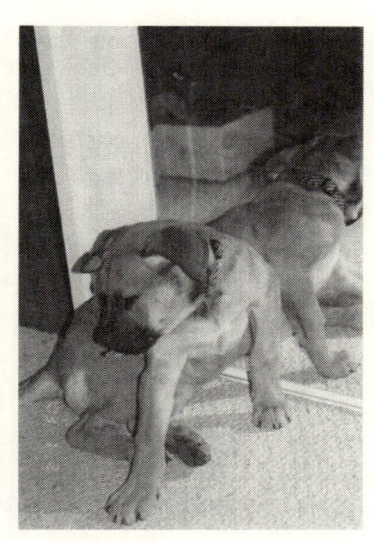

(Piggy looking in mirror)

She would swing her hips when she walked and was built real broad up front, like every woman wants to be. Her eyes were sort of sad looking, which helped her get just about everything she went after. Her floppy ears stood up when she'd lay down; this was when we could see the German shepherd in her background. Whenever someone asked about her breed, I'd tell them she was a golden Labrador/shepherd mix. This is what the Humane Society told us when she was little, and her features and coloring didn't change much at all by the time she was full grown. (It's funny that once, when I was taking a walk around the neighborhood, one of our neighbors referred to Piggy as a boxer. We always thought she had some boxer characteristics.) She weighed twenty-eight pounds at four months old. At one year, she was up to eighty-two pounds. She was just so cute I couldn't help but want to kiss her forehead every time I was near her.

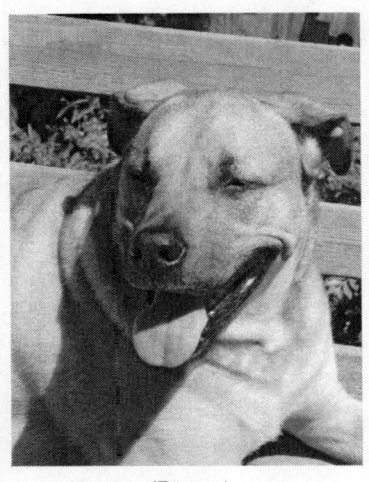

(Piggy)

Piggy was also the neighborhood watchdog. Our deck spanned the entire back of our house, which was on top of a hill. She watched the dogs in every backyard and the kids at the neighborhood day care whenever they were outside playing. There were small spaces between the fence posts that Piggy would use to play peek-a-boo with the neighbors and their dogs on a daily basis. Sometimes she'd be as still as a statue next to the fence, and I'd know she was spying on someone or the dog on the other side. Our neighborhood dogs were Roxy, a female who routinely ran the opposite side of the fence with Pigs; Charlie, a very loud beagle; and Sam, a very loud basset hound. These dogs were the primary targets for Piggy and Kermit when they spotted them in their yards from the deck. This could turn into a bark fest in a matter of minutes.

Our Piggy was a lover. She'd kiss you as long as your face was within licking range. If your face was not in reach, she'd lick you anywhere else to get attention. Even your toes would get licked whenever they were within range of her tongue. If I spent too much time writing and ignored her, she'd start whining, which sounded like she was talking to me.

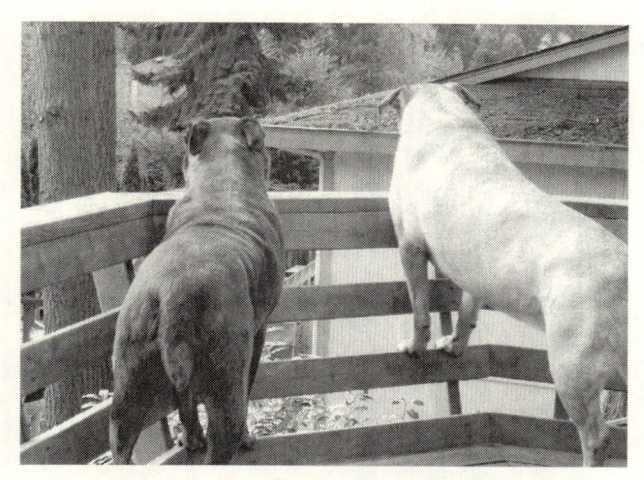

(Kermit & Piggy looking at neighbors from deck)

Ms. Piggy was your best friend when you had food. When I would be fixing the dogs dinner, Piggy staked me out. She would sit with an unmovable stare, waiting for me to put the bowls down. She and Kermit would start to eat at the same time, but Piggy almost inhaled her food. Then, if Kermit wasn't done, she'd shove him aside and eat the rest of his. This was not to say that she wasn't a sweetheart all of the time, but it was particularly evident when you had food in hand. No matter what it was, sweet or sour, fruit or vegetable, hot or cold, chicken or beef—you get the picture—she loved it. She had this sad way of looking at you like she was living in a third world country and starving. Obviously, this was how she got her name, from her love of food at a very early age. She thought a kiss should earn food, so sometimes she used it as sort of a bribe. She loved fresh, *cold* water, so I could count on a couple of kisses on my hand and a quick lick on my face every time I filled her bowl. No matter how she was feeling, she would always try to lick our faces and never acted like a drama queen. She was definitely a trouper. If her allergies were acting up, she'd just lick her paws. If she was having stomach troubles, she'd keep eating—and this goes double for the chicken and rice remedy. Over the years, we became accustomed to the signs of her not feeling good.

Ms. Piggy always picked up a squeaky toy and presented it as a gift when John got home from work. When he worked second shift overtime, he didn't get home until after midnight. Piggy would still hear him and take the rubber cookie to wait for him at the door. This might seem like such a little thing to most people, but it went on for so long. I can't be sure what she was thinking, but it was almost as if she was saying, "Thank you for coming home."

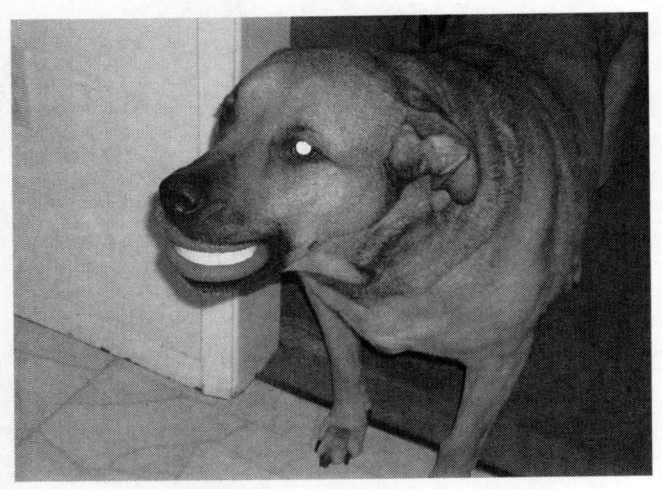

(Piggy with cookie in mouth)

Part 2
Personalities: Kermit

When I'd get out of bed or when I'd come into the living room and we'd see each other for the first time that day, Kermit would yawn and a noise that kind of sounds like "hello" would come out of his mouth. I could almost hear the words, "Good morning." When I'd get home from the

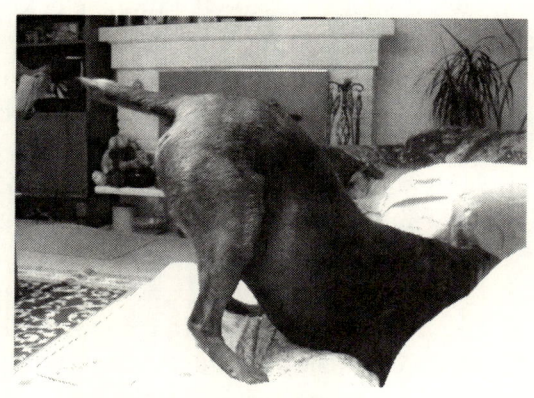

(Kermit's rear sticking in air)

gym or from shopping without the dogs, Kermit would run to the top of the stairs and give this sort of sound to Piggy that sounded like a moose. He could hear me pull in to the garage and the garage door shut. I guess this was the way he let her know I was home and she should come upstairs. Then he would do this little dance, running around from the living room to the kitchen to show how excited he was that I was home. That's my boy!

Kermit was like most men—he didn't like change of any kind. If you pushed him to try something for the first time, he'd look at you like he was saying, "Do you really want me to do that right now?" Kermit's also the "time bandit." He knows exactly when it's dinner time.

Kermit liked to rub against John after he had showered. We figured he loved the smell of Irish Spring. Even after John had dressed and sat down in his chair, Kermit would try to lick his face or rub on his arms (and legs if he was wearing shorts). He also rubbed against John's work coat; if John caught Kermit, he would tell him *no*. Fortunately, the dogs stayed upstairs with me most evenings and

John stayed down in his "man cave," so he didn't have to deal too often with Kermit's somewhat irritating habits.

I always took both dogs to the vet, even if it was only one of them who had a problem or an appointment. I couldn't imagine what the other would be thinking if left at home alone while I loaded up the other in the truck. I worried about Kermit the most, since he was the one who usually had to wait in the truck while Ms. Piggy went in for her visit. This was my way of anticipating how they might feel and trying to deal with it ahead of time. John sometimes gave me grief over this, but he'd give in to me since I did most of the driving to the vet. I was successful in including both dogs on any ride in the car, no matter whether it was to a fun place or to a visit to the vet. I'm proud of the way I've always treated my dogs with compassion. One day it was really hot and I wanted to get the dogs' nails trimmed. Since the vet's office wasn't that far away, I thought I'd take them separately so one didn't have to wait in the car while the other was inside. I put Kermit in the car and shut the door with Piggy still inside the house. Before I even got around to the driver's side car door, I heard this loud, howling cry coming from the house. It was clear this was a bad idea. And so, Piggy went too. It was kind of hard at the vet, but it was better this way than listening to Piggy cry about being left behind.

Kermit didn't play well with others. If we were taking walks, were at the dog parks, or were on a trip, he only had eyes for his sister in life, Ms. Piggy. Even when I tried to watch *Dog Whisperer with Cesar Millan* or *Cesar 911* to pick up tips on safe ways to socialize him with other dogs, my attempts bombed. I started taping these shows, but when I played them with Kermit in the room he went crazy. I have since given up on this trek, but I would love to give Cesar a challenge. Kermit would probably have to go to his dog rehab center for treatment, and I'm not sure I could give him up for that long.

Chapter Eight

Health Problems

Piggy had always been a high-maintenance dog, but until recently nothing was life threatening. She had allergies. With dogs, these manifest themselves in a reaction, many times with a rash on their tummies or even tenderness in the underside of the paws. We first noticed this problem with Piggy when we discovered her licking her paws excessively. There were many days when I had to soak her feet in a special solution if she had played in the yard very long. She was just like a human, because her reactions appeared primarily in the spring and summer when pollen was in the air. I tend to believe the allergy diagnosis as opposed to depression, which has also been linked to excessive paw licking in dogs.

I always talked to Piggy and Kermit as if they were regular people; however, until you start seeing health and other problems manifest themselves in them the same way as a human, it doesn't hit home just how much they are like us. Dogs' symptoms are treated with some of the same medications too. For example, Piggy took Benadryl every day for watery eyes, sneezing, and itchy paws during the high pollen seasons. Check with your veterinarian before administering this to your pet, because dosage is based on weight for most animals.

You may want to consider giving your animal an antacid for stomach acid or gas. This is particularly important if you decide to follow our recommended grain-free/vegetable diet. Again, you should check with your vet before deciding on a brand or dosage. Vegetables are hard to digest for some dogs and can sometimes cause gas, just like in humans. This is especially true with broccoli or cauliflower, so I tended to stay clear of these except for a treat now and then. I would occasionally toss the dogs a few pieces if I was eating those vegetables steamed for dinner. I did this with green beans, too, when I was having them for my meal. I slept closer to the dogs than John did, so I was the one to suffer the consequences (gas). Because of this, I tended to watch this part of their diet a little closer than he did or I'd feed them some during the day so the gas would be pretty much gone by bedtime.

I recommend trying Bonine for motion sickness for any trip taking an hour or more. The dosage is 25 mg for every fifty pounds—but, again, you should check with your vet for your individual animal. During one of our first three-hour drives to the beach, Piggy got motion sickness in the Jeep. I decided not to take any chances on this happening with Kermit, so he was required to take it just like Piggy. It worked out okay, because it made them sleepy and they would take a nap during the drive to wherever we were going that weekend.

Throughout the years, we dealt with the dogs' minor health problems, such as a cyst between the toes in both dogs, glaucoma in one of Piggy's eyes, and a benign cyst on Kermit's eyelid. Here are a few simple tips on how we spotted these problems and how to catch them early:

- Cysts between dogs' toes are not uncommon. Most of these are benign. Whenever we spotted even a slight limp, we'd check for splinters, a rock stuck in their pads, or a growth. Even though most of these are benign, we always chose to have them removed to relieve discomfort.
- We discovered a cloudy cover on one of Piggy's eyes, so we had her checked out by a specialist. It was the beginning of glaucoma. From that time on, we had to put prednisone drops in both eyes every day. She never complained about it, but the specialist told us that without treatment this would have caused her to have really bad headaches, similar to a human's migraine.
- One of the most prevalent problems for our dogs were fatty tumors. These, too, are normally benign, but the vet will have

to take a sample to look at the cells before telling you the diagnosis. Kermit had a fatty tumor the size of a grapefruit close to his private parts. He urinated to one side, that's how big it was. We've since had it removed. Doc Annie said it was so large "it deserved its own zip code." Thank goodness it was benign.

Each time we faced these issues, we were scared of what we might find out. But the sooner you get them checked out, the better. Although the remedies for the ailments would oftentimes be kind of expensive, nothing was too good for our Kermit or Piggy. We always managed to cover the expenses somehow. I will always remember Doc Annie telling us she wanted us to adopt her. That made us feel good about how we were taking care of our dogs, although we were still short of angelic, I suppose.

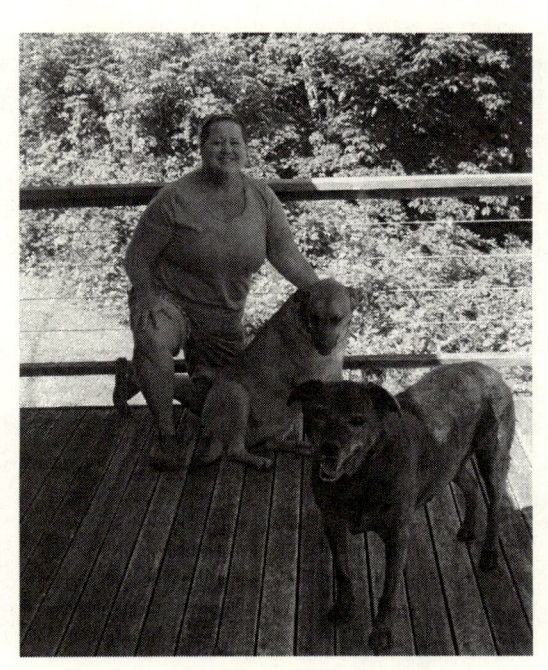

(Pennye with dogs)

Chapter Nine

The Diagnosis

On December 3, 2009, we received the worst news possible. I remember it like it was yesterday. Piggy had not been her normal self for a couple of days. She played around with her food as opposed to her usual habit of scarfing it down like it was the best meal she'd ever eaten. I might have waited a couple more days to take her to the veterinarian, but John insisted I take his princess the next day. I felt like this was jumping the gun a little, but it turned out this was not the case. I thought maybe we should just try some chicken and rice. I'm so glad I took her.

I called first thing in the morning for an appointment that day. Doc Annie must have realized Piggy's lymph nodes were swollen when she first saw her, because she went straight for the exam behind her front legs. She confirmed all four lymph nodes behind her legs were swollen. Doc Annie looked up at me teary eyed and said she was 90 percent sure it was lymphoma and shook her head. *This can't be happening*, I thought and started crying. *How am I going to tell John that his little girl has cancer?* Piggy lay there wearing her Santa's helper scarf. She was only seven years old, and Christmas was only weeks away.

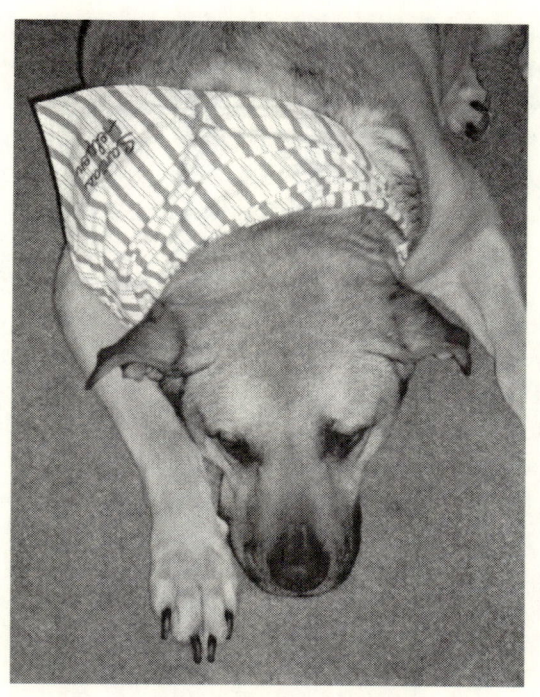

(Piggy with Santa scarf)

John was at work, so I was at the veterinarian's office alone. I kept thinking, *Maybe there is another reason for the swelling. Cancer can't be taking our precious princess. She doesn't deserve to die.* Doc Annie used a long needle to draw some of the fluids out of one of Piggy's front lymph nodes. She said she'd send it to the lab and we would find out the results within a couple of days. I hugged Doc Annie. She said how sorry she was and told me she would call as soon as possible with the test results. The tests would basically be the confirmation of the diagnosis. I knew in my heart Doc Annie wouldn't have even mentioned lymphoma if she wasn't 99 percent sure, and she wouldn't have wanted to give me this information over the phone. She knew I would need time to accept this. I could have kicked myself for not noticing the enlarged lymph nodes sooner. Piggy was so chubby—at over one hundred pounds—and this allowed me to sort of forgive myself for not seeing it sooner. I wouldn't have been expected to notice this without trained eyes or hands. We briefly went over some treatment scenarios. In the back of my mind I was thinking, *How in the world are we going to afford any of these?*

The folks at Chambers Creek Vet are just awesome. We wouldn't have made it through this ordeal without their loving care and support. This might sound weird since I'm talking about our dog, but there was just something about Piggy that made everyone love her more than just a normal dog.

I had found a part-time job and had to go to work after taking Piggy to the vet, so I couldn't stay with her. I called on my break, when I knew John would be home from work, to deliver the horrible news. I hated to do it over the phone, but John would usually be in bed by the time I got off work so waiting wasn't a good solution either. I needed to know if Piggy ate her dinner, and only John would know this. I could hear him gasp and start to cry over the phone line. He said, "Well, maybe it won't be lymphoma." I wanted to feel more positive, but if he had seen the look on Doc Annie's face after she'd examined Piggy earlier in the day, he would know—as I did—that the tests were just a confirmation of what we already knew.

> Lymphoma is a form of cancer that primarily begins in the lymph nodes but can be found in other organs. It's one of the most common tumors in dogs. This disease usually presents itself in dogs between the ages of six to nine. It is more prominent in certain breeds. Additional information can be found at http://www.wearethecure.org/lymphoma. Without treatment, dogs usually die in four to six weeks.

John and I had both lost our fathers to cancer. My dad had died more than fifteen years ago, so I had come to terms with it long before this happened. But John's dad had died only a couple of years ago. His dad's illness had been very hard on him and the rest of his family. I knew Piggy's diagnosis was going to hit him like a lead balloon.

When I arrived home from work that night, John was sitting in the living room with one hand on Piggy, crying his eyes out. I didn't know what to do. I was sad, too, but one of us had to be strong. The next day, I told one of the girls at work about his reaction. She said, "Tell him to suck it up and start researching this disease on the Internet." She mentioned we should consider an all-natural diet. I had been so wrapped up in the diagnosis and wondering how we would pay for the treatment, I had overlooked an obvious massive source of information.

We cancelled all of our unnecessary expenses to trim our monthly budget. (This was not a lot, because we were already doing this since I'd lost my job.) We determined what money we had available on our credit cards and if we could make the monthly minimum payments. I was only working part time because of my wrist injury and was still waiting to see if it improved enough so I could go back to work full time. Two days later, the diagnosis had been confirmed and Piggy was getting her first chemo injection. John and I were learning about the protocols for treating dogs with lymphoma as well as other cancers.

I was working part time at REI (Recreational Equipment, Inc.) as a seasonal employee in the membership services department. I knew about REI's reputation as an employee-owned and employee-oriented company, but I truly experienced it firsthand. When I mentioned I might need to take a day or two off, they were very understanding. Each day Rhonda, my supervisor, would ask how Piggy was doing. (Later the next year, she even e-mailed me to ask about her condition.) This was the kind of employer I wanted to be working for as opposed to my previous employer, who I have already described and will not dwell on any longer.

Although I was bringing in some income, it wasn't even close to my previous salary and the position would soon be ending. Let's call this another blessing in disguise. Even though we needed the money, Piggy needed almost round-the-clock care and monitoring so it would have been really hard for me to work and be able to take care of her too. I didn't know what we were going to do or how we would pay the bills. John was good at living on a strict budget, so I turned it all over to him after the diagnosis was confirmed. I knew this would be in the back of his mind every time he saw Piggy from now on.

Next began a massive research effort to identify anything else we might need to know. Even with the World Wide Web at our fingertips, the lack of information available for canine cancer treatment was surprising. We turned to information on lymphoma treatment as it related to humans with this illness. This was overwhelming. We'd have to trim even more from our budget to afford the recommended diet of high protein and fat. We're talking chicken, beef, and pork in addition to an expensive grain-free kibble. Even after all this, there was no question that we'd start the treatment as soon as possible.

The day after we received the confirmation that it was lymphoma was terrible. We couldn't stop crying, and John didn't want to miss work. As he left, I told him I'd call after Piggy's appointment for her blood work. An hour later, I was off to the veterinarian's office with Piggy and Kermit in tow. It was seven o'clock in the morning—time for the first of many blood tests. Doc Annie had to be sure Piggy's immune system could handle the first intravenous chemo treatment. This disease acts fast, and the blood tests would also help determine what stage the cancer was in. Next, Chambers Creek Vet reviewed our options and shared some great articles on the treatments available along with side effects and the recommended basic diet composition.

The next thing Doc Annie said almost turned me to stone. She told me Piggy would last only a month if we decided against the chemotherapy treatment, so we didn't have much time to think about it. This was confirmed in the research we were able to find. I'm the kind of person that would like to analyze a decision of this magnitude, but there wasn't time. This became even more real to us as we saw her weight drop drastically in the week following the diagnosis. She dropped from 104 to 94 pounds in only a few days. She wouldn't eat and did nothing but sleep and look up at us with bloodshot eyes, like she had the flu. We tried her favorite food, chicken and rice, but she still didn't eat.

We received an estimate of the cost for a six-month treatment plan and were told we'd need to pay at least 50 percent up front. The estimate was about six thousand dollars. I had recently opened up a dental/medical charge card for some dental work and discovered it could be used at most veterinarian offices too. All charges over one thousand dollars would be interest free for a year. So we at least had an initial payment plan, and we had hope that I would be bringing in more income in the near future.

After the blood results came back the next day, I took Piggy for the first of what would be the toughest days during the next six months of her life. This was just the beginning of our fight to save our four-legged daughter's life. Doc Annie didn't give us much reason to get our hopes up. She said even with treatment, we should hope for only an extra year with Piggy. I kept telling John how Piggy could sense how we felt and we should only think positively so she would get discouraging vibes from us. Every day I had to encourage him to think positive. If it hasn't become totally obvious by this point, we loved her so much. It was getting harder for me to keep up my positive attitude. Most people don't understand a love this strong for a pet, so I found it hard to talk to my friends about it. I prayed and even spoke in the front of church on Sunday, asking everyone else to say a prayer for Piggy.

Piggy received her first intravenous chemo treatment two days after her diagnosis. She was so good about lying still and, as usual, stayed one of the favorites at Chambers Creek. Jan was usually at the front desk. Her nickname for Piggy was Mama. Piggy's weight continued to drop to an all-time low of seventy-nine pounds. Then miraculously in week three, she gained almost two pounds.

Piggy slowly but surely was responding to the treatment. This is important because if she didn't show immediate improvement, we didn't have much hope for another treatment program with any history of success. We fine-tuned our special diet, and her appetite improved. Our hopes and prayers for her to go into remission seemed like they were going to come true. Then came week number three. The work-up this week called for a blood panel to assure she was stable for the addition of the drug Cytoxan. This was a powerful drug that was administered at home along with prednisone and furosemide (Lasix).

We tried to do everything possible to make Piggy comfortable. John purchased a twin-size memory foam mattress for both dogs to sleep on. This was mainly for Piggy, but we needed enough room for her and Kermit to sleep side by side.

By this time, I had decided it was my destiny to do everything possible to save Ms. Piggy's life and to help others going through the same ordeal with their pets. In doing this, Kermit could continue to have a playmate for life and we would have our princess. I didn't know what Kermit would do without her or what John would do without his princess.

Chapter Ten

Understanding the Treatment

With a diagnosis early the first week of December, Piggy was scheduled to begin her series of chemotherapy treatments on Friday, December 4, 2009. We were given a twenty-five-week course of treatment that reflected what kind of drugs she would receive each week. The schedule was based on the "Madison Protocol." (If you enter this description into your search engine, you will get over one million results. I recommend putting in the time to find the best and most up-to-date site if you are trying to find information about this for your pet.) Finally, we were finding out what we needed to know. This is a special chemotherapy used to treat canine lymphoma. It's odd that they have uncovered the cause of the lymphoma virus in felines and cows but not in people or canines.

> The *Wisconsin Lymphoma Protocol* (also known as the *Wisconsin Protocol*, the *Madison Wisconsin Protocol* and other mixed terms) is a shorter, but dose-intense chemotherapy regimen currently popular with oncologists as the primary canine lymphoma treatment, with a success rate of around 91%, according to Dr. Mike Richards, DVM. This chemotherapy protocol uses vincristine, doxorubicin,

cyclophosphamide, and/or 1-asparagnase by IV, along with prednisone and/or cyclophosphamide orally.

Whatever the case, keep in mind that each chemotherapy cycle can take between 2–3 hours to complete; side effects vary but can include vomiting, diarrhea, and appetite loss (but not hair loss, unlike in humans) and during treatment it is not uncommon for dosages and drugs to change according to effectiveness. For this reason it's best to have an oncologist on your dog's health team with plenty of chemotherapy experience.[1]

There has been an enormous amount of research progress, even since December 2009. It is very important to diagnose this disease early to prevent its spread to internal organs. Although I'm certainly not a veterinarian, I consider myself well educated on this disease when it comes to canines. I also know how food and supplements can affect the success of the treatment.

What is the life expectancy with treatment?

It is impossible to predict how long your pet will live. Unfortunately, most dogs with lymphoma are not cured of the disease. However, with treatment 80–90% of dogs will achieve remission. With the use of the 25 week University of Wisconsin-Madison protocol, average first remission lasts 10–14 months, with 20% 2 year survival. When a patient's lymphoma relapses, chemotherapy may be restarted and the majority of dogs (70–80%) will achieve a second remission. Generally the second remission is shorter than the first. Sometimes a third, fourth, and even fifth remission can be achieved, but each is generally shorter than the last as the cancer cells become resistant to the chemotherapy just as bacteria become resistant to antibiotics.[2]

Piggy Pooh started her chemotherapy the first week of December 2009 and ended it the last week of May 2010. Blood tests were done every other Wednesday and the medication was administered on the following Thursday, assuming she was strong enough to handle it based on the results of the blood tests for that week. Thankfully, there were a few bye weeks within the schedule when she had a break. (We lived for these weeks.) These gave her body time to recuperate and prepare for the next round of drugs. We were very lucky that her immune system passed the tests every time. I'm not sure how we would have held up if her system had declined and we'd had to postpone that week's treatment.

We had faith in Doc Annie. She was very knowledgeable and would recommend only the best. She had known Piggy since she was eight weeks old, and she loved her almost as much as we did. She knew how much it meant to us to save Piggy. We depended on her to let us know when it came to the point that Pigs was suffering and it was in her best interest to let her go. When I said this to Doc Annie, she told me we would know.

The first month included almost daily doses of prednisone to help build up her immune system. (We began these the day after the diagnosis.) Then the fight was on. In a matter of just a couple of days, we had armed ourselves with all of the information we could access. I do have to admit that John did the lion's share of the research. However, I had the responsibility of taking Piggy to all of her appointments and doing all of the grocery shopping. Initially, we used the food processor to cut the veggies into small pieces for Piggy's meals. After a while, we discovered that the cooked vegetables should be put through the blender, which made them easier to digest. Together, John and I learned the best way to prepare her food and took turns cooking the vegetables and chicken we added to their nighttime meals.

Chapter Eleven

The Diet and Supplements

  We examined all of the food, biscuits, and treats that were part of the dogs' daily diets. Piggy began to drop weight at an alarming rate as her body tried to fight off the cancer and accept the chemotherapy. All of the research we were able to find stressed a high-protein and high-fat diet for canines with this illness. Absolutely no grains, sugars, or starches! These, we were told, feed the cancerous tumors. We threw away all of the dry dog food, a gigantic box of name-brand biscuits, and countless treats that contained primarily grains or carbohydrates. If we didn't have the nutritional information for something, we'd call the toll-free number on the packaging or look for it online. If you are health conscious about your pet's diet, you may be surprised and depressed about what is in the foods most people feed their animals.

  We searched for grain-free dry food to use as a dietary base. We discovered there were a few out there, but we couldn't find them in our local store. Then one evening on my way home from work, I stopped at the feed store in downtown Sumner, Washington. The manager was kind enough to answer all of my questions as I searched for a grain-free food with a high percentage of protein. He gave me free samples of a grain-free dog food called Taste of the Wild. There was salmon, fowl/duck, bison, and a couple more varieties.

> My suggestion when selecting food or treats is grain-free, high-protein (18 percent or more) kibble (ours was closer to 28 percent), probiotics, fish oil (500 mg or more, depending on dog's size). Stick with American made & packaged. Canned pumpkin helps with upset stomachs.

When I brought the samples home, I was excited to try them out. I was anxious to see if Piggy would eat them or at least be able to keep some down. Her appetite was just not anywhere close to what it should be and nothing like it was before she had been diagnosed. Doc Annie was concerned about her ability to maintain her weight or at least lose as little as possible during the next six months. Luckily, Piggy was a little on the heavy side when she got sick, so she could stand to lose a little weight and still be okay. Kermit and Piggy loved the samples I fed to them and ate the kibble without any water or anything.

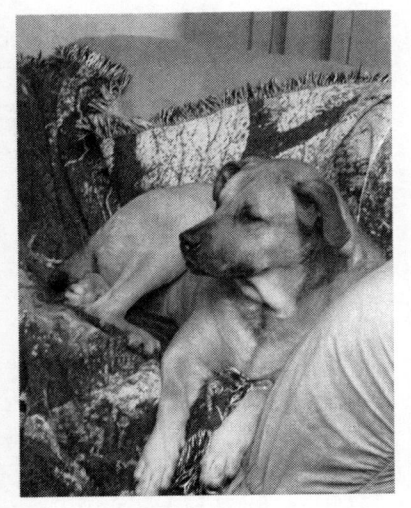

(Piggy in chair)

Next, I set out to add more fresh vegetables to their meals. I began with carrots, garlic, zucchini, leeks, sweet onions, and broccoli. First, the veggies were put through the food processor, and then they were mixed together and slowly cooked in chicken broth (preferably organic and low sodium). Little by little, we discovered other veggies to add, such as fresh mushrooms, radishes, green beans, cauliflower, and spinach. We tried to alternate what we included depending on what was in season and therefore more cost effective. This mixture added to the Taste of the Wild dry food along with cut up cooked chicken or beef became the mainstay of the dogs' diets. Details on the entire recipe, best vegetables to use, and how to prepare the food are contained at the end of this book.

The dogs digested this food fairly quickly. What I'm getting at is they were often hungry again very, very early in the morning. For a while, we were serving cut up pieces of pork roast for breakfast.

We could buy pork roasts in a bulk package of four at a time at the local warehouse club, so it sounds more expensive than it really was. Once the treatment was over and Ms. Piggy had regained her weight and strength, we had to find another breakfast. Fortunately, she was back to living up to her name. We served a vitamin-packed meat roll designed for dogs after discovering how much they liked it. These are available in most pet stores and some grocery stores. They are fresh and refrigerated.

One of the supplements we included in the daily regiment was glucosamine chews for their joint health. Bigger breed dogs are much more likely to develop various cancers, hip dysplasia,

> Glucosamine/chondroitin sulfate is great for joint health in humans and dogs. These supplements are particularly good for large dog breeds. After our dog developed arthritis at age five, we utilized the prescription Rimadyl for joint pain. Ask your veterinarian for more information.

and other joint problems, so these supplements don't necessarily tie to the lymphoma diagnosis. The supplement we used was Joint MAX and contained not only glucosamine but chondroitin sulfate, manganese, vitamin C and E, grape seed extract, zinc, alpha lipoic acid, selenium, citrus bioflavonoids, plus traces of a few other ingredients. These are effective for arthritis and joint and skin health in addition to being a powerful antioxidant. A couple of other naturopathic ways I suggest to help with overworked joints and sore muscles include laser therapy and battery-operated massage tools.

We also added approximately 1800 mg of fish oil to the dogs' food by squeezing the oil from a couple of gel tabs into their kibble every night. They loved this because it was fish flavored. This supplement has about the same benefit for humans as it does for dogs and is good for your heart.

When fighting an illness like cancer, it's important to get as much dietary nutrition as possible. Some of our methods and ingredients might seem a little excessive, but they were necessary. We always made sure the flavor was there, because taste was essential to ensuring our pets ate well during any healing process—especially when Piggy was going through chemotherapy. Remember that anytime your pet has trouble keeping food down, chicken and rice is the best remedy.

Pennye A. Lentes

We kept a supply of this in the fridge the entire time Piggy was going through chemo. Again, I didn't want Kermit to feel left out or get treated different from Piggy if at all possible, so anytime it was in my control he had the same thing as she did, such as the chicken and rice or pork for breakfast. The only time I strayed from this was I did end up leaving him at home when Piggy was getting chemo treatments. At times it's dangerous for healthy pets to be close during this procedure.

Chapter Twelve

Chemotherapy

Piggy's first week of chemotherapy consisted of receiving an intravenous drug called L-asparaginase (Elspar). The procedure took only about thirty minutes, and I had to wait for her in the lobby area. After she was done, she came out with her signature smile, her abnormally long tongue hanging out. That made me feel better, because I thought at least it seemed like it didn't hurt her. We also gave her Prednisone twice a day for seven days to boost her immune system. This continued until week four, when she began to get sick to her stomach and very tired.

During the first three weeks of chemotherapy, Piggy lost over 15 percent of her body weight. She started out weighing 104 pounds, which was a little overweight for her body style and size. Her extra weight was yet another one of our blessings in disguise. Luckily, we had some room to play with. But when she reached 85 pounds, she looked thin and frail. Her skin was sagging, and we started getting scared and wondering if we had made the right decision to put her through chemo. Doc Annie assured us that Piggy was okay and her weight loss was slowing down. Doc Annie just smiled and said, "She's at her fighting weight."

Piggy was responding well to the treatment. Her lymph nodes were beginning to shrink. If your pet has cancer in another area of the body, your vet might need to take x-rays to tell if they are responding to the treatment. It's very important to make sure the cancer is responding to the type of treatment. If not, there are alternate types of treatment. We felt good that Piggy Pooh was showing almost immediate improvement and was in remission by week four. This made us feel a little better. The thought of her wasting away over the next few months was devastating.

Week two of chemo called for an oral medication that we were required to pick up at our local drug store. This drug, Cytoxan, was so toxic that the pharmacy didn't even order it until a day prior to pick-up time. We were to give her five tables (50 mg each) as one dose. The tablets had to be handled with rubber gloves. This drug is normally given at home along with something to calm the stomach to reduce the possibility of any nausea and vomiting. While Cytoxan can kill both healthy and cancerous cells, it has a greater effect on cells that are multiplying rapidly. Generally, cancer cells multiply more rapidly than regular healthy cells, so cancer cells are more affected by the drug.

Chambers Creek wanted to do an ultrasound during this first round of Cytoxan, so I took the tablets with us to the vet's office one Wednesday morning. Prior to administering the drug, Doc Annie wanted to make sure the cancer hadn't spread to any of Piggy's internal organs. This can be compared to types of cancer in humans that metastasize in the liver, which is not a good sign and may require a change in the treatment. Piggy couldn't have anything in her stomach for the ultrasound, so they had to wait to give her the Cytoxan until after the procedure. We warned them that they would need to make sure she had something in her stomach before she took the pills. They said they'd give her some canned all-natural food. Piggy got very sick after this round of Cytoxan, and we dreaded future treatments with it. We knew there was a good reason for taking it, but it was still really hard on Piggy's system.

Cytoxan is a wicked drug. The precautions surrounding acquiring it and handling it should tell you how toxic it is. When I picked Piggy up after work later that day, she looked kind of weak. The techs at Chambers Creek assured me she had been able to keep down the dog food meatballs they had used to give her the Cytoxan. They mentioned I might want to have her urinate before taking her home, because she hadn't gone out for a while. The next thing they said really got to me: "Make sure you take her to the special side of the building to urinate."

I then realized the degree of toxicity of this drug, because she couldn't even urinate around other dogs for two days after taking it. We had to keep her apart from Kermit for forty-eight hours. This was tough. Kermit didn't really understand what was going on or why they had to be separated for two days. *Oh well*, I thought. *I know it's for the greater good.* I hoped Piggy would tell Kermit what was going on so he didn't think he was missing out on anything.

By the time we got home that night—a week before Christmas—Piggy wasn't responding well to her first dose of Cytoxan. She started vomiting, so I was up all night long with her. Between cleaning up the mess and trying to get her to keep down food or water, I was getting really scared. I thought she would surely die with her head on my lap. Each time she drank or ate anything, she vomited. By the next morning, she could barely get around. I rushed her to Chambers Creek as soon as they opened. They said she was dehydrated and would need to be on intravenous fluids for most of the day. I went to pick her up at the end of the day, and she seemed much better. John took off work on Friday to take care of her. Then we both nursed her back to health that weekend with small servings of chicken and rice and plenty of water.

We decided we needed to have a different plan in place before Piggy was scheduled to receive Cytoxan again. It became the most dreaded drug of the entire protocol. I hated the thought of her having to take this again, but it was in the schedule three more times.

By now you must be wondering why in the world Doc Annie would prescribe Cytoxan if it caused such horrible side effects. I did too, so I did an enormous amount of research on the drug. It turns out Cytoxan is also used for human cancers. It is approved to treat breast and ovarian cancer, lymphomas, leukemia, and others in humans. It's also prescribed for "minimal change" nephrotic syndrome in children (a kidney disorder) when other treatments have failed. With such broad spectrum use in humans, I had to trust it was a necessary part of the treatment. I tried to compare it to having to eat yogurt when you're on antibiotics because some antibiotics kill the good and bad bacteria. Yogurt puts the good back in.

I usually had a knack for finding the silver lining when the going got tough, but it was getting more difficult each day to find anything that even resembled a silver lining. I continued to search for the blessings in disguise. As it was, every time Piggy had to go to the vet, Kermit sat in the car or at home alone. It looked like he was saying, "I never get to go." If he only knew what awaited her every visit: blood tests, ultrasounds, or IV chemotherapy.

Weeks four, five, and six went by slowly but without any major problems. We still had to use chicken and rice for meals because of the effect of the chemo drugs. By week seven, it was time for another dose of Cytoxan. We discussed several things to change this time so she wouldn't get so sick. We gave her something to settle her stomach and made sure to have plenty of chicken and rice on hand. Kermit stayed downstairs and Ms. Piggy upstairs for the next forty-eight hours. John and I took turns with both of them for the required two days of separation.

We had given the dogs chicken and rice as a remedy in the past, but it was usually when Piggy had trouble with her bowels. Kermit never had trouble with his stomach, so this was kind of a fringe benefit for him for just being around during the dark times. He deserved something special. He saw Piggy getting special treatment, but I doubt he knew what was going on. Maybe he did. Maybe they communicated in dog language and Piggy told him she was very sick. (She did lick him in the ear all of the time.) This could be when she broke the news to him.

Fortunately, Pigs rebounded from the weeks that included the Cytoxan treatment. But the separation time made me give some serious thought to how Kermit would do without Piggy to keep him active and playful. I was worried he would give up on life without her.

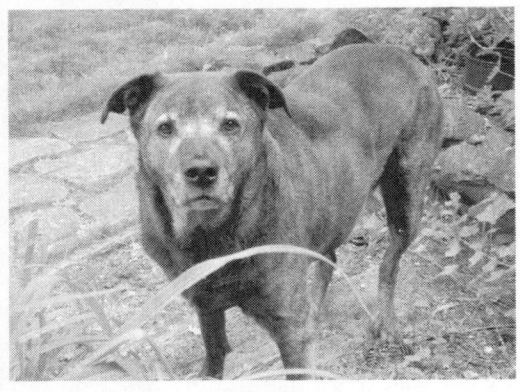

(Kermit)

I decided to go back to thinking positively. Piggy was going to be that one-in-a-million dog who recovered. If any dog could it, it would be her.

Week twenty-five was the final week of chemo. It took about one and a half hours to administer the final intravenous dose of doxorubicin. Piggy was in full remission with no more treatments necessary. We planned for a visit to the beach in June, after she'd had a few weeks to rest. She looked great and was eating again. Both her and Kermit liked the all-natural, grain-free diet. We were vigilant with everything both Piggy and Kermit ate.

Chapter Thirteen

Another Minor Health Crisis

In January 2011, Piggy started limping on her back right leg. She had slipped a little during a ride in the car earlier that day, but I couldn't imagine any permanent damage could have come from it. A couple of days and a visit to Chambers Creek later, we discovered she had torn her anterior cruciate ligament (ACL). They recommended surgery and warned us about the detection of hip dysplasia. We were told when one knee goes, chances are the other will go because she would rely heavily on the good leg after surgery. We didn't like this idea, so we decided to limit her activity and give her something for the pain along with anti-inflammatory meds. In a way, this was a good diagnosis; we had been so scared she had come out of remission and the cancer was in her bones.

There were a couple of alternative treatments that sounded promising. The first we tried was acupuncture. Acupuncture was supposed to help with pain and promote healing to the injured area. The cost was seventy-five dollars per treatment. We saw some improvement after the first treatment so decided to try it again two weeks later. Unfortunately, Piggy flinched every time a needle went in. This was heartbreaking. It almost felt like abuse, so that was the final treatment. I do think this promoted some initial healing. Had she accepted it better, we would have continued.

Another alternative treatment being used was lasers. There were only three veterinarians in the State of Washington that used it. Chambers Creek was one of them. There was still that fear in the back of our minds that if she came out of remission after receiving the laser, we would kick ourselves forever. We decided against pursuing this option.

Twelve long months later and we were still nursing this injury, hoping some miraculous cure would present itself—and hoping it would be one that didn't cost a fortune. Some recent research had revealed surgery performed on dogs as test subjects. The doctors replaced their tendons with ones from another animal, like a pig or something compatible. The recuperation period was short. This looked like a promising option if it would become available. We just wanted Piggy to be happy and live a quality life for what was left of it, with Kermit at her side.

We researched stem cell therapy for her hind leg and for the arthritis in her front shoulders. After extensive communication with specialists, we were told that type of invasive surgery could throw her out of remission so we tabled that idea. We limited her use of the steps and tried to keep her from jumping up and down on the deck benches. We also tried to revise her diet to help her lose a little weight. She had put on about fifteen pounds of what she had lost during her chemo, which was good and a little bad. The docs said that less weight on her legs would help both her front shoulders and her back leg. It was hard to find a common ground, because her exercise was limited so she really didn't burn off a lot of calories.

Chapter Fourteen

Admitting Defeat

In August 2012, we received a perfect report card for Piggy from her quarterly blood tests. It was raspberry season, and Piggy followed me through the patch for a bite here and there. Kermit was lying in the sandbox and not really interested in the berries. We had a bumper crop of raspberries that year. While I was harvesting them, I'd throw a berry to each dog. Kermit spit his out, so he didn't get any more. As I picked more berries, I found that my bowl didn't seem to get full. I realized Piggy had been sneaking bites out of the bowl. I hoped she wouldn't get a stomachache. At the end of the day, she was fine and there were plenty of berries for all of us.

We handled Piggy's pulled ACL because we knew how much worse it could be. More stem cell research success stories are being documented every day. I hope to give a portion of the proceeds from the purchases of this book to

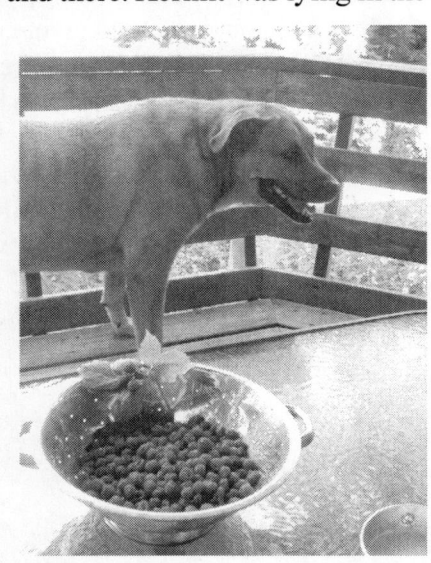

(Piggy with raspberries)

assist with this research in addition to helping our local Humane Society, where our story began.

Again, many thanks to everyone responsible for Piggy's three years of remission. Whether it was God or another higher being, we received more good fortune than we thought ever possible. The average remission for dogs is twelve to fourteen months. We made it to three years; I still just can't believe it!

I reflect back on the first half of 2010, I hope that somehow Piggy let Kermit know what was going on. He needed to know it was serious and it didn't have anything to do with him or how he lived his life.

I hope by now you love Piggy and her story as much as we do. I have documented almost all of her life through pictures, so we can look back years from now and remember the good times.

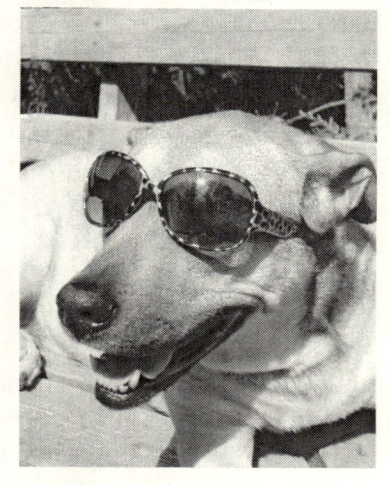

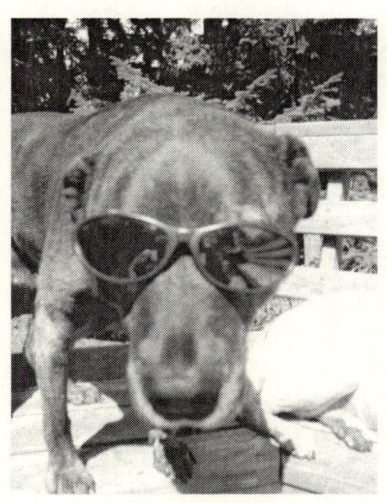

(Piggy with sunglasses)

(Kermit with sunglasses)

John said Piggy always squinted in the sun, so I decided to see if she liked sunglasses. She did. Kermit only kept his on long enough for me to get one shot off, but it's still a great pic, don't you think?

If you are dealing with any kind of canine cancer, I recommend finding an oncologist or a vet like Doc Annie who is highly educated in the treatment of this disease or a specialist in oncology. Enlisting the help of a specialist can lead to having your pet around for a lot longer than anticipated and with a higher quality of life. We lucked out that Piggy's regular vet, Doc Annie, was very educated in oncology.

I hope the information I've included will help others facing the same problems to realize there is always hope. I have a desire to travel around the United States giving seminars (or host online webinars) on how to treat a sick canine and providing suggestions on dealing with other health problems. Even though I'm not professionally trained in animal care, I have information that comes from the heart. While some of these options might take time and patience, they are worth it. We are comfident our ability to have Ms. Piggy in our lives for three years after her diagnosis can be attributed to the immediate change in diet. This includes many of the items I have discussed like the grain free kibble and treats, nutritional supplements and the tender loving care of a veterinarian like Doc Annie.

Piggy had just turned seven when she was diagnosed. The dogs were going to turn ten years old on October 1, 2012.

My mother-in-law, Betty, came for a visit during September 2012. We planned to go to the coast for a few days with the dogs. John had rented a house in Westport right on the beach.

I picked Betty up from the airport, and we headed home. John was still at work, but Betty and I started packing things for the trip. We started out early the next morning with the Explorer packed full. We were going to stay a week, and it looked like good weather ahead. We got to the house and unloaded things. The dogs were thirsty, so we set up a place in the kitchen with their water and food bowls. We headed to the beach and let the dogs run.

On our first night, I fed the dogs their special diet. For some reason, Piggy didn't want to eat. I started to freak out. John told me not to worry and reminded me that they were always picky eaters when we were someplace other than home. The week went by fast, and we had a lot of fun. However, Piggy still wasn't eating much, and she had vomited a couple of times. We gave her something for her stomach. The last day, we packed up and headed home.

On the way home, Piggy vomited and had diarrhea. We had to stop a couple of times for her to use the bathroom and for us to clean up the car. When we got home she seemed a little better, but she still didn't want to eat much. The next day, I took Betty to the airport. I took Piggy to her oncologist as soon as I returned home.

In Remission

Piggy wasn't eating or drinking, and I was freaking out. The oncologist immediately took her in the back and started an IV to rehydrate her. I waited in one of the rooms for some news. Dr. Gillings came in and said she didn't detect any abnormalities in Piggy's lymph nodes, but she said Piggy was very dehydrated. She wanted to run some tests, so I gave her the go-ahead to find out what was wrong. When I told her we had been at the beach for the past week, she suggested maybe Piggy ate something like a dead fish and had picked up a bacterial infection. I prayed that was all it was.

A couple of days and a couple of thousand dollars later, we learned Piggy had come out of remission and the cancer was in her stomach. We decided to transfer her back to Chambers Creek and try another round of chemo, hoping she would respond as quickly as she had before. We decided it would be well worth it, even if we could get only another couple of years with her.

Unfortunately, luck wasn't on our side this time. Piggy went downhill fast. She wouldn't eat, so I had to feed her liquid food with a large syringe. I also learned how to insert the IV so I could hydrate her at home. I dreaded the thought of her having to stay at the vet overnight.

We made a bed for her downstairs with a bunch of blankets. John and I took turns sleeping and lying with her. At this point in time, we just didn't want to give up. John went to work, and I was home with her all day. She could barely walk to make it outside to urinate. She had very little food in her and didn't have any interest in eating. Another two or three days went by like this, and we knew it was time to give up the fight.

On Saturday, October 6, the weather was great so we decided to take Piggy and Kermit for a ride through Point Defiance Park. Piggy seemed like she felt good with her head sticking out of the window, catching the air and smiling with her tongue hanging out.

When we got home, John and I smiled at each other and thought maybe she was getting better. This feeling was short-lived. As soon as we got home, she went downhill fast. I think it was maybe like the burst of energy that people often get right before the end. We had scheduled for Doc Annie to come to our house and put Piggy to sleep so she could pass peacefully. But after what we had just experienced on the ride through the park, we thought maybe we had jumped the gun and Piggy just needed more time to get better. We canceled the appointment.

Three days later, on Tuesday, October 9, Piggy could barely walk. She made it down to her favorite place underneath the evergreen and collapsed. I had to almost carry her back up to the door to the basement. I called and rescheduled her last appointment. Doc Annie came. We kissed Piggy good-bye while crying and holding different parts of her. Then she was gone. Kermit was in the basement while this was going on. All of a sudden we heard this bloodcurdling cry. It was coming from Kermit.

We had her remains cremated. They are in a wooden box that is displayed on our mantel along with our favorite pictures of her and other mementos: her Vikings collar, the blue leash, and a few special rocks from the beach.

I know some people who read this won't understand, but this was the kind of love that a person rarely has a chance to have. A year and a half later, we still have trouble talking about her.

Kermit was a healthy, almost twelve-year-old mastiff mix. He was hooked on television. His favorite show was called *Dogs in the City*, but he loved anything with animals and would be glued to the *Dog Whisperer with Cesar Millan*. Sometimes he was just a statue while watching, and other times he would go crazy, barking constantly. He'd had surgery for a large fatty tumor on his stomach, but other than that he had been fine. I knew he missed Piggy as much as we did. He would still look for her at her favorite spots when he'd go into the backyard. Unfortunately, his time to reunite with Piggy came before we were ready to let go of him; though, in reality, I don't think we would ever have been ready.

Kermit was diagnosed two months ago with cancer. It was in his spleen. After several more tests, we were told it had metastasized to his liver. We had his spleen and one of the larger nodules on his liver removed. After his many staples were removed, we took him for a final trip to the beach. He was slow but still wanted to fetch his toy. We were amazed and excited about having him in our lives for a few months longer. Kermit passed on August 17, and I know he joined Ms. Piggy in dog heaven.

I know they are both angels watching over us and playing in the clouds. We miss you!

All-Natural Diet Preparation

This makes about eight helpings. One batch usually lasts about four days for two large dogs. (Our dogs each weighed about ninety-five pounds.) You don't want to make more that this amount, because it can go bad just like fresh vegetables. (If you're cooking for only one dog, cut the ingredient portions in half.)

Dinner
Dissolve chicken bouillon in about five cups of water. Put the first group of vegetables through a food processer and cook (simmer) for about fifteen minutes:

3 chicken bouillon cubes
2 zucchinis (medium size)
3 radishes (average size)
1 cup green beans (these can be fresh or frozen)
1/2 cup frozen spinach (or 2 cups of fresh spinach)
1 1/2 cups fresh carrots

I cook the following in the microwave and add it during the blender phase:
1 medium sweet potato or butternut squash

After the mixture and sweet potato cools down, blend ingredients together using a food processor or blender. This makes it easier for the dogs to digest. Warm up enough for one meal every night before mixing it with the dog's grain-free kibble. Add diced cooked chicken. It's best to make only enough chicken and vegetables for two to three days so the mixture retains its flavor.

Each night I would add the fish oil from two gel tabs (1200 to 1500 mg total) to each dog's meal along with a crumbled glucosamine treat. (Piggy also received Rimadyl and Proin for pain and incontinence.)

(I have tried making this ahead and freezing it, but it's not quite as good. I might try canning it so I can take it on the road with me.)

Breakfast
For breakfast, each dog received about 2 ounces of Fresh Pet beef meat and vegetable roll. (Piggy would also get a few more glucosamine treats to help with her arthritis.)

Chicken and Rice (for those upset stomach days)
The amount of rice will depend on the size of your pet and what you consider a serving. For a ninety-five-pound dog, cook approximately 1 1/2 cups of rice and 1 cup of diced chicken breast.

Travel Tips

1. Schedule a veterinarian visit prior to departure to ensure overall health and current vaccinations. Ask for a health certificate and vaccination records, especially if you're traveling out of state.
2. Make sure your pet's identification tags are up-to-date and legible. Also, be sure his rabies tag and vaccination are current.
3. Include your destination address and/or phone number on your pet's tags and cage/crate (if applicable).
4. Remember to pack water to prevent dehydration. The Handi-Drink works extremely well and allows your pet to drink from it. To help ensure convenient feedings, bring along a collapsible food bowl.
5. Pack all medications and supplements to avoid missed doses.
6. Pack a first aid kit to ensure readiness in the event of an injury or medical emergency.
7. Exercise your pet prior to departure. A tired pet is typically much more amenable to travel. Also, bring a lead or harness to allow exercise during pit stops.
8. Feed your pet at least four hours prior to departure to prevent car sickness. If the trip is going to be long, feed a smaller amount than normal at least two hours before you leave.
9. Use a travel remedy, if necessary. If your pet is extremely anxious about travel, try a soothing nonprescription product like our Ultra-Calm, Rescue Remedy, or Comfort Zone Spray with D.A.P (Dog Appeasing Pheromone).
10. Trim toenails to prevent snags and injury, especially if your pet will travel in a cage or crate.
11. Cover your car seats with our seat covers to keep them clean and free of hair shed on your trip.
12. Know travel rules and restrictions, especially if you will be traveling on an airplane.

Bibliography

1. Reexam,Lymphoma*Info.net*, copyright 2009–2014, CanineLymphoma.net, last updated 9/12/14, http://www.lymphomainfo.net/blog/general-lymphoma-blogs/canine-lymphoma-treatment.
2. CanineLymphoma.net, copyright 2009–2014, http://www.caninelymphoma.net/canine-lymphoma-treatment-options.php.

Other Sites Used for Gaining Information but Not Specifically Quoted:

Institute for Integrative Nutrition
http://www.integrativenutrition.com/go/education
The basic nutrition section was used to investigate the vegetables for the special diet.

Premium Pet Supplements
3688 Research Way, Suite 1
Carson City, Nevada 89706
Copyright 2012–2014
http://www.dogcancer.net/success.html

Care must be used when referencing websites with recommendations that are primarily intended for human use. We utilized many sites that were really for humans with cancer. We took some of the basic information and used it to help Ms. Piggy. For example, sugars, grains, and carbohydrates feed tumors. We took this information and used it to examine some of the foods and treats our dogs ate. Unfortunately, most of the items we regularly fed them contained a high percentage of these items. This led us to change their entire diets and start preparing the new all-natural with veggies and grain-free diet described above.

In Remission

Pennye Lentes lives in the Pacific Northwest with her husband and two dogs, Kermit and Ms. Piggy (and Monty, a 6 ft. python). After 20 years in marketing, she's become an advocate for the care and diet necessary to keep dogs healthy and in remission.

CPSIA information can be obtained
at www.ICGtesting.com
Printed in the USA
FSOW01n0530020115
4282FS